Student Learning G

Pharmacologic Basis of Nursing Practice

4th edition

Julia B. Freeman Clark, PhD

Sherry F. Queener, PhD

Virginia Burke Karb, PhD, RN

Prepared by Linda Wendling
Editorial Consultant
St. Louis, Missouri

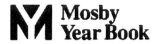 **Mosby**
Year Book

St. Louis Baltimore Boston Chicago London Philadelphia Sydney Toronto

Editor: Robin Carter

Design and Layout: Ken Wendling

Cover Design: Gail Morey Hudson

Project Manager: Carol Sullivan Wiseman

Production Editor: Shannon Canty

Printed in the United States of America.

CHAPTER 1

General Principles of Drug Action

BUBBLES

The answer to each of the clues in this puzzle is a five-letter word related to principles of drug action. Enter each word into the grid by placing its first letter in the center of the correspondingly numbered bubble, and the remaining letters in the four outer spaces, proceeding either clockwise (+) or counterclockwise (-) as indicated by the sign following the clue. It's up to you to determine where the outer four letters begin in each bubble. The first three are done for you. Good luck!

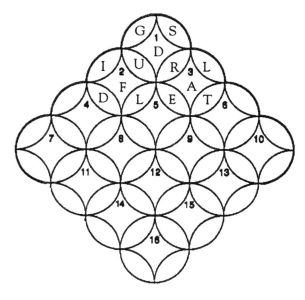

1. _____ can be excreted unchanged in the urine. (+)
2. Antacids alter pH of stomach _____. (-)
3. Drugs may chemically _____ body fluids or cell membranes. (+)
4. Drug interactions that alter cell membranes are usually _____ based. (+)
5. 3 main routes of drug elimination: liver, kidney, and _____. (-)
6. Disintegrators allow a tablet to absorb _____ and break apart. (-)
7. _____ injections are absorbed slowly. (-)
8. TI is the _____ of lethal dose in 50% of the population to the dose effective in 50%. (+)
9. In hypertension therapy, several drugs amplify the action of the others to _____ blood pressure. (+)
10. Most important site for biotransformation of drugs. (+)
11. The time between drug administration and a response is called the _____ of action. (+)
12. _____-genic means "caused by a drug." (-)
13. Type III drug reaction: "_____ sickness." (-)

14. Enteral drugs may have binders, fillers, or dis_____rators. (+)
15. Therapeutic chemicals (+)
16. Unpredictable drug reactions are of two _____: idiosyncratic and allergic. (+)

BLOCKOUT!

Hidden in the box below are five words related to principles of drug action discussed in this chapter. Each word is divided into five letters, each in only one block in each column. Cross out each block as you make it part of a word that solves one of the numbered clues below, and write the word itself in the correspondingly numbered blank. The first word is done for you.

E	L	A	S	D
R	S	E	E	M
B	P	P	G	A
U	D	A	I	D
S	A	E	M	E

17. EDEMA

18. _____

19. _____

20. _____

21. _____

17. Symptom of anaphylaxis.
18. Alcohol + drugs = _____ heart rate.
19. Damaged tissue may do this.
20. Act or consumption of drug therapy.
21. Succinylcholine can prevent muscle _____ during surgery.

1

Legal Implications of Drug Therapy

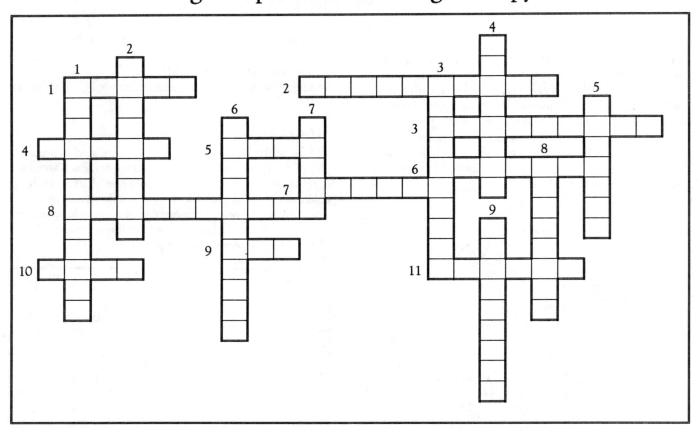

ACROSS

1. The ancient Egyptians used parts of the _____ plant to relieve pain.
2. Another name for physical addiction.
3. Drugs with a high potential for abuse and no accepted medical use.
4. The name given to a drug by its manufacturer.
5. Aspirin tablets are examples of drugs taken via the _____ route.
6. The name applied to a drug, no matter who manufactures or sells it.
7. Drugs that are not profitable to develop.
8. Drugs in Schedule G are _____ drugs.
9. In the DESI rating system, if a qualification to the use of a drug is made, it is rated "Effective _____."
10. After the Kefauver-Harris Amendment, the FDA contracted the National Research Council to evaluate all drugs being sold in the US through this project.
11. The law that designated certain drugs as legend drugs was the _____-Humphrey Amendment.

DOWN

1. *The United States _____.*
2. An example of a drug chemically synthesized.
3. Controlled drugs whose use is restricted to specific conditions described by law.
4. _____ bark was used to relieve malarial symptoms.
5. Nonharmful, noneffective substance.
6. A _____ experiment is one in which neither patient nor medical personnel know which patients are receiving the test drug and which are receiving the placebo.
7. Bovine insulin is standardized on the basis of the amount of the preparation required to reduce the _____ sugar by a specific amount.
8. Laws like the Harrison Act were designed to _____ use or distribution of drugs.
9. Drugs used primarily for relief of pain but also possessing significant psychotropic activity; identified in Canada by letter *N* on label.

Application of the Nursing Process to Drug Therapy

CODE BREAKER

Below is a familiar message from Chapter 3. We have simply substituted each letter of the alphabet with a different one. Letter substitutions remain constant throughout. For instance, if **z** = **r**, then it will equal **r** *everywhere* it pops up in this puzzle. As you translate each letter code, write the real letter being represented underneath its code letter every time you encounter it. One word has been done for you.

CAT ROUT ZOPACB DR EZMP

____ _____ _____ __ ____

GEFOJOBCZGCODJ: CAT

_____: ____

~~ZOPAC~~ EZMP, CAT ZOPAC ZDMCT,

<u>RIGHT</u> ____, ___ _____ _____,

CAT ZOPAC EDBT, CAT ZOPAC

____ _____ ____, ___ _____

COFT, GJS CAT ZOPAC XGCOTJC!

____, ___ ___ ____ _____!

TOSSED-WORD PUZZLE

Unscramble the terms to reveal strategies for helping patients take medications as ordered. Then unscramble the boxed letters to answer the riddle.

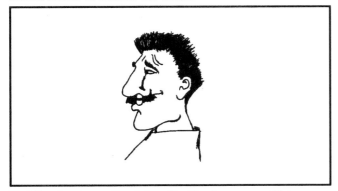

Riddle: Annie realized that Paul's clever use of his new capsules indicated a problem with

_ _ _ _ _ _ _ _ _ _.

a. r e d a c l a n ☐ _ ☐ _ ☐ _ _ _

b. c r o o l d e c d o s p u c
_ _ _ ☐ _ _ _ _ ☐ _ _ ☐

c. r a l a m ☐ _ _ _ ☐

d. h e c a n g n i o d e s
☐ _ _ _ _ _ ☐ _ _ _ _

HIDDEN AGENDA

Terms relating to the nursing process and drug therapy are hidden in the grid below. They may appear vertically, horizontally, diagonally, left-to-right, or right-to-left. First solve the clues below to fill in the blanks. Then locate each in the grid by either highlighting or circling it. The first one has been done for you.

a	s	s	e	s	s	m	e	n	t	x
g	c	a	v	e	p	o	o	r	d	n
n	o	c	a	s	s	m	o	r	p	g
i	n	f	l	n	y	r	o	u	r	y
y	f	l	u	c	h	c	e	v	a	g
r	u	l	a	s	e	a	m	e	c	l
r	s	o	t	r	a	d	d	i	t	e
a	e	d	i	a	g	n	o	s	i	s
c	d	r	o	m	s	a	n	t	c	e
p	l	a	n	n	i	n	g	r	e	m

<u>assessment</u> _____ _____

_____ _____

_____ _____

_____ _____

_____

Over-the-Counter Drugs and Self-Medication

BUBBLES

The answer to each of the clues in this puzzle is a five-letter word related to OTC drugs and self medication. Enter each word into the grid by placing its first letter in the center of the correspondingly numbered bubble, and the remaining letters in the four outer spaces, proceeding either clockwise (+) or counterclockwise (-) as indicated by the sign following the clue. It's up to you to determine where the outer four letters begin in each bubble. The first three are done for you. Good luck!

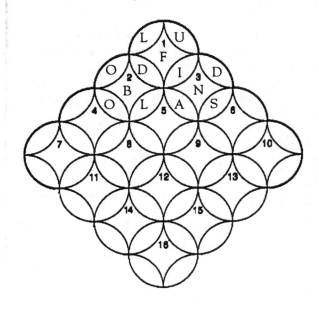

Clues

1. An expectorant should, by one definition, help in the expulsion of _____ from lungs and bronchial passages.(+)
2. Aspirin can cause the loss of _____ in the stool.(+)
3. Abbrev. nonsteroidal antiinflammatory drug.(+)
4. In "rebound congestion," congestion after a drug's effects have worn off may be _____ than before treatment.(+)
5. Most OTC cold remedies contain a drug to relieve sinus and _____ congestion.(+)
6. Antibacterial soaps or antiseptic solutions are usually not necessary, since infectious bacteria don't normally _____ in acne.(+)
7. Codeine can _____ psychologic and physical dependence.(+)
8. Bulk producers are probably no more effective at suppressing appetite than is drinking _____ before meals.(+)

9. A suncreen with an SPF of 8 will protect 8 _____ as long as unprotected skin exposure.(+)
10. OTC bulk producers may _____ a laxative effect.(-)
11. Diphenhydramine is an example of an antihistamine approved for use as a _____ aid.(+)
12. Diphenhydramine is considered the _____ useful of the approved antitussive drugs.(+)
13. Comedones consist of a mixture of _____ and epithelial cells.(+)
14. Dextromethorphan side effects include GI _____.(+)
15. Large doses of codeine may _____ constipation, nausea, and drowsiness.(+)
16. Aspirin can cause the stomach or intestinal lining to _____.

BLOCKERS

Hidden in the box below are five words related to OTC drugs and self-medication. Each word is divided into five parts and concealed sequentially from left to right in consecutive columns. For example, one of the words is **MUCUS**, with the letter **M** in the first column, **U** in the second, **C** in the third, **U** in the fourth, and **S** in the fifth. Identify, on the blanks below, each word hidden in the accompanying box. Cross out squares as you find each word, because each will be used only once.

T	U̶	O	N	L
A	E	C̶	N	S̶
M̶	O	U	T	E
W	O	N	U̶	H
R	M	I	A	D

17. MUCUS _____

18. _____

19. _____

20. _____

21. _____

CHAPTER 5

Care of the Poisoned Patient

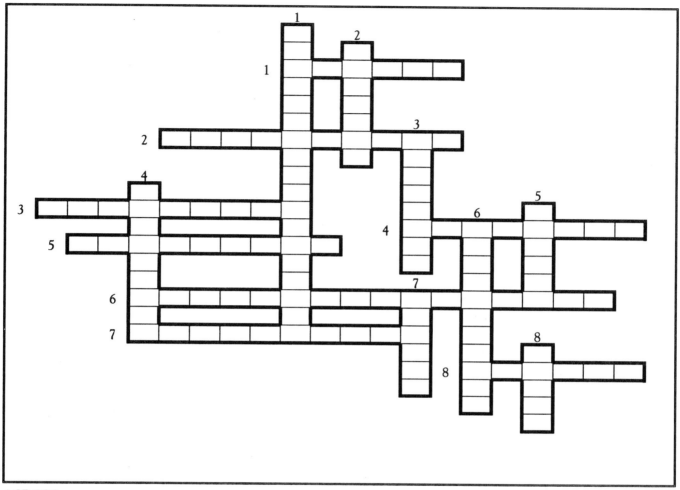

ACROSS

1. Ipecac syrup is used to _____ vomiting.
2. _____ are the final common treatment to reduce absorption of poisons from the GI tract.
3. Computerized database on most medicines and consumer products with potential danger of poison.
4. Activated _____ absorbs a number of chemicals, preventing their absorption into the body.
5. Ataxia may indicate poisoning by one of the sedative-_____.
6. It is common to flush poison from the _____ tract.
7. Drowsiness or coma may indicate poisoning by a _____.
8. The emetic of choice.

DOWN

1. The study of care of the poisoned patient.
2. Antidote for lead poisoning.
3. Induction of vomiting should not be used when time is _____.
4. Vomiting is not indicated when the vomitus can be damaging to the _____.
5. Toxicokinetics deals with the _____ of a poison in the patient as a function of time.
6. Poisoning by local _____ can cause convulsions or twitching.
7. The stomach is emptied by _____ or gastric lavage.
8. Dialysis is used in cases of extreme poisoning or _____ failure.

CHAPTER 6

Drug Administration

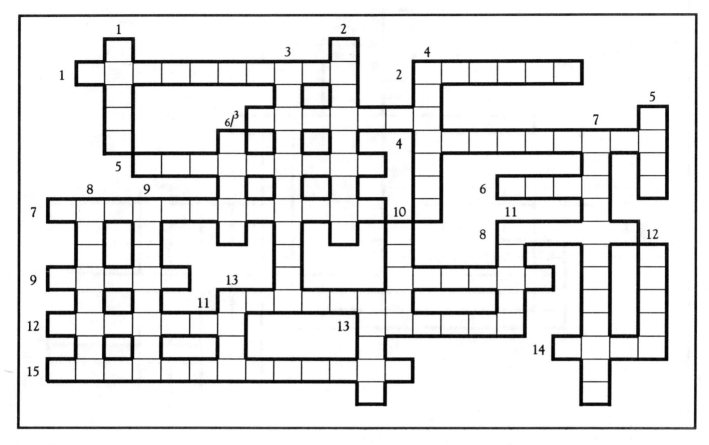

ACROSS

1. Assessment data is both _____ and objective.
2. IM site for up to 5 ml of drug is the _____-gluteal site.
3. Pruritis.
4. Parenteral doseform.
5. The vastus _____ site is found in the thigh.
6. Venous access device: the implantable _____.
7. _____ injection delivers below skin with a 23- or 25-gauge needle.
8. A topical dose form.
9. In the _____ system, each patient unit is supplied with large-quantity drug containers.
10. _____ tablets are dissolved between cheek and gum.
11. Drug form for the eye: the sustained _____-insert.
12. Drug form dissolved in the mouth.
13. Drug form dissolved in the mouth.
14. IV drugs may be administered via a heparin _____.
15. Chronologic age may not match the _____ age.

DOWN

1. _____-inhaler.
2. Method (e.g., Z-track _____).
3. Injection made just below the epidermis.
4. A douche is an example of a _____ drug.
5. Nitroglycerin ointment doses are ordered by the _____.
6. Most forms in patient records are _____ documents.
7. Emergency infusion in children.
8. "_____" means each dose is individually wrapped, labeled, and supplied in quantities to last 24 hours.
9. Children's comprehension is _____ until early teens.
10. Not all skin preparations may be applied _____-ally.
11. _____ a drug in suspension form before pouring.
12. In Z-_____ technique, pull skin taut to one side before inserting the needle.
13. Inhalation drugs are given via _____-iratory system.
14. Give liquids that stain the teeth via a _____.

Calculating Drug Dosages

MATCHING

Identify the correct meaning of the pharmaceutical abbreviations on the left by writing the correct letter in the blank.

_____ 1. o.u.   a. every hour

_____ 2. q.h.   b. both eyes

_____ 3. stat.   c. immediately

_____ 4. p.r.n.   d. by mouth

_____ 5. p.o.   e. according to circumstances

CONVERSIONS BETWEEN APOTHECARIES' AND METRIC SYSTEMS

Calculate the answers to these problems.

6. gr 1/100 = _____ mg

COMPUTING ORAL DOSAGES

Calculate the following for tablets, capsules, or liquids:

7. Desired: Aspirin gr x q 4 hr
   Available: Aspirin 0.3 gm/tablet

8. Desired: Chloral hydrate syrup gr viiss TID
   Available: Chloral hydrate syrup 10% solution

COMPUTING PARENTERAL DOSAGES

9. Desired: Morphine sulfate 10 mg
   Available: Morphine sulfate 16 mg/cc

10. Desired: Penicillin G 400,000 U IM
    Available: Penicillin G 1,000,000 U in 5 ml

COMPUTING IV INFUSION RATES AND TIMES

11. The physician orders 1000 ml 5% D/W to be administered in 4 hours. Drop factor is 10 gtts/ml. Calculate:

    a. The number of minutes the medication is to flow
    b. The number of milliliters the patient will receive per minute
    c. The number of drops the patient will receive per minute

12. Give 1000 ml 5% D/W at 30 gtts/min. Drop factor is 15 gtt/ml. Calculate:

    a. The total number of gtts to be given
    b. The total number of minutes to flow
    c. The total time for infusion in hours and minutes

13. Give 400 ml Ringer's Lactate in 3 hours. The drop factor is 15 gtts/ml. Calculate:

    a. Total number of minutes to flow
    b. Number ml patient will receive/min
    c. Number drops/min

CALCULATING PEDIATRIC DOSAGES

Calculate the following dosages for children:

Adult Dose	Age	Data for Children Weight (lb)	Height (in)	Children's Dosage Clark	Young	BSA
14. Atropine Sulfate gr 1.150	18 mo	25	32	_____	_____	_____
15. Aminophylline 0.5 gm	6 yr	38	42	_____	_____	_____
16. Gentamycin 80 mg	22 mo	28	38	_____	_____	_____

Introduction to Neuropharmacology

BLOCKERS

Hidden in each box are eight words divided into eight parts and concealed sequentially from left to right. Using the clues, fill in the corresponding blanks to identify each word hidden in the accompanying box. Each square will be used only once. The first clue is done for you.

e	y	en	p	p	l	i	s
s	e	c	a	ph	a	e	e
h	s	u	i	r	d	i	s
r	f	f	i	o	m	k	c
c	o	n	e	c	e	e	l
v	o	r	e	y	n	a	ng
p	e	s	z	n	er	ff	a
a	e	r	m	t	t	e	t

1. e f f e r e n t

2. _____

3. _____

4. _____

5. _____

6. _____

7. _____

8. _____

1. _____ neurons relay data *from* CNS.
2. Sensory receptors send signals via _____ neuronal pathways.
3. Neurotransmitters are stored in _____ in the terminal.
4. The space between the neuron and the cell with which the neuron is communicating is the _____ cleft.
5. Acetylcholine and norepinephrine are used in the _____ nervous system.
6. Acetylcholine is synthesized by choline acetylase from choline and an acetate molecule activated by _____.
7. Epinephrine is one of the neuro-_____ because it is released into the blood to produce effects at distant sites.

8. When norepinephrine is taken back up into the neuron from which it was released, the process is called _____.

n	h	p	o	a	g	i	ry
de	p	l	b	er	c	or	e
o	d	i	n	s	i	g	y
t	o	g	i	n	a	o	c
a	e	o	l	t	er	v	or
r	h	re	r	i	i	t	e
ch	e	e	a	la	t	t	c
in	c	g	u	er	t	i	ic

9. _____

10. _____

11. _____

12. _____

13. _____

14. _____

15. _____

16. _____

9. The _____ (sympathetic) nervous system.
10. The _____ (parasympathetic) nervous system.
11. Activation of cholinergic and adrenergic receptors produces _____ responses.
12. Parasympathetic control of the cardiovascular system is primarily that of a reflex _____ system.
13. The preganglionic neurons of the adrenergic nervous system arise from the _____ and lumbar regions of the spinal cord.
14. The parasympathetic nervous system has dominant control over "_____" processes.
15. Transmitters like GABA and glycine are _____ rather than excitatory.
16. Neurons respond to inhibitory neurotransmitters by developing a more _____ resting potential with a decreased likelihood of firing.

CHAPTER 9
Mechanisms of Cholinergic Control

TOSSED-WORD PUZZLE

Unscramble the terms below, using their clues to help you, and write them in the blanks. Then unscramble the boxed letters to fill in the blank under the riddle.

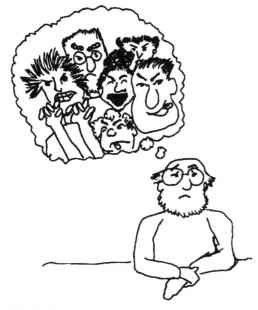

RIDDLE: In pharmacology, unlike "real life," this can be an ally. An __ __ __ __ __ __ __ __ __ __ __ __ __

1. C R A I N M U C I S
__ __ □ __ __ __ __ □ __

2. N O T E C I N I
□ __ __ __ □ __ __ __

3. R A R E C U B O U I N T
□ __ __ □ __ __ __ □ __ __ __

4. T H A N C I R O C L I N G E I
□ □ __ __ __ __ __ __ __ __ __ □ __ __

CLUES:
1. _____ (parasympathetic postganglionic) receptors
2. Laboratory agent that mimics the effects of acetylcholine at the skeletal muscle and ganglionic receptors
3. Blocks receptors for acetylcholine at neuromuscular junction causing muscular relaxation or paralysis
4. Drugs that block the action of acetylcholine by occupying the receptor and preventing cholinergic action

TRUE OR FALSE   Circle the correct answer.

T F 6. In overdose, atropine may cause malaise and hallucinations.

T F 7. Scopolamine and atropine are often referred to as belladonna alkaloids.

T F 8. Tubocurarine primarily blocks the receptors for acetylcholine at the neuromuscular junction.

T F 9. Acetylcholine is a commonly used therapeutic agent because it produces many responses and rapidly degrades in the blood.

T F 10. Restoration of muscle tone in patients with myasthenia gravis or in surgical patients treated with tubocurarine is one of the therapeutic uses of cholinomimetic drugs.

T F 11. Clinical uses of each class of acetylcholine antagonists are interchangeable.

T F 12. Certain tremors caused by Parkinson's disease, other diseases, and by certain drugs are called extrapyramidal motor effects.

T F 13. Blockage of secretions is a therapeutic use of muscarinic receptor antagonists.

T F 14. Muscarinic receptor antagonists also dilate the eye (mydriasis) and paralyze accommodation.

T F 15. Atropine is administered to decrease the heart rate by antagonizing the acetylcholine released by the vagus nerve at the atrioventricular node of the heart.

MATCHING   Match the drug with its class or indication.

____16. Physostigmine (Eserine), pyridostigmine (Mestinon), and neostigmine (Prostigmin)

____17. Demecarium (Humorsol), echothiophate (Phospholine), and isofluorphate (Floropryl).

____18. Carbachol (Carbacel), pilocarpine (Pilocar)

____19. Bethanechol (Urecholine)

____20. Pralidoxime (PAM)

A. irreversible acetylcholinesterase inhibitors
B. only systemic direct-acting cholinomimetic
C. ophthalmic direct-acting cholinomimetic drugs
D. antidote for irreversible acetylcholinesterase inhibitor poisoning
E. reversible acetylcholinesterase inhibitors

CHAPTER 10

Mechanisms of Adrenergic Control

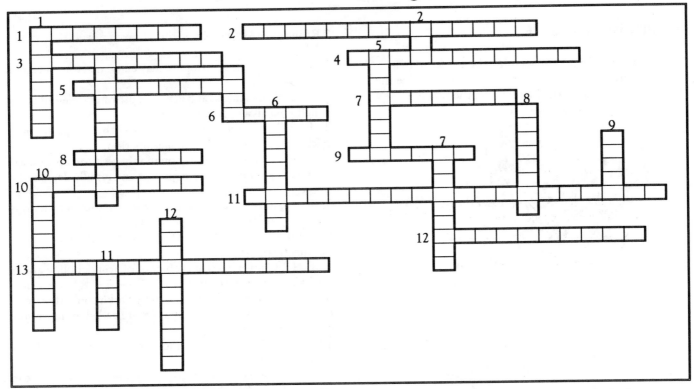

ACROSS

1. _____ is derived from the amino acid tyrosine and is the chemical precursor of norepinephrine.

2. Dopamine, norepinephrine, and epinephrine are naturally occurring _____ .

3. _____ has both alpha- and beta-antagonist action.

4. First beta blocker approved for use in U.S.

5. Propranolol is effective in treating _____ headaches although the mechanisms involved are not clear.

6. _____ receptors are receptors for which norepinephrine and epinephrine are equally potent, but isoproterenol is less potent.

7. Guanethidine and reserpine act by depleting norepinephrine from peripheral _____ .

8. Catecholamines are ineffective when taken _____ because they are rapidly destroyed in the GI tract or by the liver.

9. Blockade of beta-2 receptors limits bronchiole dilation, therefore avoid in _____ patients.

10. Cardioselective antagonists (beta-1 selective antagonists) include _____ and metoprolol.

11. Clonidine and methyldopa decrease sympathetic tone mainly through an action in the _____ .

12. _____ researched how epinephrine caused glycogenolysis in the 1950s.

13. In the autonomic nervous system, _____ is the sympathetic, postganglionic neurotransmitter.

DOWN

1. Responses to activation of beta-2 receptors include _____ of the bronchioles.

2. Cyclic _____ is the key to intracellular action of epinephrine.

3. Local anesthetics have a longer duration of action when _____ is injected to slow systemic absorption.

4. _____ receptors are receptors for which isoproterenol is more potent than or as potent as epinephrine or norepinephrine.

5. Chronic hypertension and _____ disease are indications for reserpine and guanethidine.

6. Alpha-2 receptors are found on _____, smooth muscle or the blood vessels that determine blood pressure.

7. Dilation of the pupil.

8. Most prominent systemic effect of alpha-1 receptor activation is an _____ in blood pressure.

9. Responses to activation of beta-1 receptors include stimulation of the _____ .

10. Nadolol, labetolol, penbutolol, and pindolol are classified as nonselective beta-receptor _____ .

11. Epinephrine and isoproterenol are _____ .

12. Neurohormone released from adrenal medulla in reaction to stress.

CHAPTER 11

Drugs to Control Muscle Tone

SHORT ANSWER

Complete the following statements:

1. _____ is a disease in which the skeletal muscles quickly show weakness and become fatigued.

2. _____ (ptosis) is an early sign of myasthenia gravis.

3. In myasthenia gravis, what results if the intercostal muscles and the diaphragm become affected?

_____

4. What is the basic defect in myasthenia gravis?

_____

_____

5. What causes an autoimmune disease?

_____

_____

_____

6. What causes myasthenia gravis?

_____

_____

_____

7. What are the contraindications of the anticholinesterase drugs?

_____

_____

_____

8. Describe the mechanism of action for the neuromuscular blocking agents.

_____

_____

_____

DRUG PROFILES

Match the drug to the appropriate drug profile.

_____9. Ambenonium (Mytelase)

_____10. Pyridostigmine (Mestinon)

_____11. Tubocurarine (Curare)

_____12. Atracurium (Tracrium)

_____13. Doxacurium (Nuromax)

_____14. Pipecuronium bromide (Ardvan)

A. A nondepolarizing neuromuscular blocking agent used to produce muscle relaxation during surgery or electroconvulsive shock therapy. Also reduces muscle spasm in tetanus, and allows controlled ventilation.

B. Drug of choice for myasthenia gravis treatment.

C. New long-acting nondepolarizing muscle relaxant, has desirable feature for coronary disease patients.

D. Nonbromide salt used to treat myasthenia gravis, drug of choice for patients allergic to bromides.

E. Nondepolarizing muscle relaxant. Shorter duration than tubocurarine, does not produce cardiovascular side effects.

F. Nondepolarizing muscle relaxant with long duration of action, used for procedures lasting 90 minutes or longer. Has no vagal blocking action to cause tachycardia.

CHAPTER 12

Drugs Affecting the Eye

BUBBLES

The answer to each of the clues in this puzzle is a five-letter word related to drugs affecting the eye. Enter each word into the grid by placing its first letter in the center of the correspondingly numbered bubble, and the remaining letters in the four outer spaces, *proceeding clockwise*. It's up to you to determine where the outer four letters begin in each bubble. Good luck!

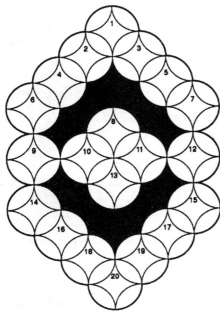

1. Miosis refers to a constricted_____and is achieved by stimulating muscarinic receptors of the sphincter muscles.

2. Mydriasis refers to a dilated pupil and is achieved by blocking muscarinic receptors of the sphincter muscles or stimulating_____receptors of the dilator muscles.

3. Glaucoma is the increase in IOP as a result of_____accumulation between lens and cornea.

4. Since atropine is applied for 3 days,_____children for systemic reactions, discontinue application if any reactions appear.

5. Chronic (open-   )_____glaucoma is the most common form of glaucoma and has a gradual onset.

6. Scopolamine, a potent mydriatic, is used like atropine but cycloplegia_____for only 3 instead of 6 days.

7._____laser treatment may be the preferred first treatment for glaucoma.

8. In the eye, newly synthesized prostaglandins_____a miosis that resists the mydriatic action of atropine.

9. Sphincter and ciliary muscles_____when anticholinergic drugs are instilled into the eye to hasten the healing of inflammatory conditions.

10. Among the unpleasant side effects of carbonic anhydrase inhibitors are appetite loss, gastrointestinal_____, lethargy, and depression.

11. Cholinomimetic drugs in chronic glaucoma increase the area of the anterior chamber to improve the uptake of the aqueous_____.

12. Phenylephrine and hydroxyamphetamine are in the adrenergic drug_____.

13. Children are the most_____to systemic toxicity from ophthalmic drugs.

14. Cycloplegia refers to the paralysis of the ciliary muscles by_____that block muscarinic receptors.

15. The_____advantage of beta blockers is that neither pupil size nor reactivity to light is altered.

16. The autonomic nervous system plays a major role in controlling the amount of_____entering the eye and in focusing images.

17. Glycerin, mannitol, urea, and isosorbide are osmotic agents used to_____IOP before surgery or as an emergency treatment of acute glaucoma.

18. Betaxolol, levobunol, and timolol may produce systemic side effects; most commonly a decrease in_____rate and fall in blood pressure.

19. Carbonic anhydrase inhibitors may be_____to glaucoma therapy when the combination of weak miotic, epinephrine, and timolol does not lower intraocular pressure.

20. Most beta blockers produce corneal anesthesia, which_____to corneal damage.

Drugs Affecting the Gastrointestinal Tract

HIDDEN AGENDA

Terms relating to drugs affecting the gastrointestinal tract are hidden in the grid below. They may appear vertically, horizontally, diagonally, left-to-right, or right-to-left. First solve the clues below, then locate each in the grid by either highlighting or circling it.

```
B E T H A N E C H O L A P C F
S D O I N G L M H C G E O A G
T P C S T I M U L A N T S N S
C R L M A E I F F Q U I C T U
A N T I C H O L I N E R G I C
N O S M I U B Y L S B C R H R
N P T I D P L O C T A L M I A
A I A T S J Y I O L R M N S L
B O I O Y W W U S A S N O T F
I I M I S O P R O S T O L A A
N D M L G N R L H O F X Z M T
O S I E N E G I O M I E R I E
I O R H O R J M C O D E I N E
D A L A C T U L O S E R O E H
P E S C O P O L A M I N E S O
M E T O C L O P R A M I D E L
```

1. _____ (Urecholine) is the only direct-acting cholinomimetic drug with sufficient tissue specificity to be administered systemically.

2. _____ (Reglan) is a dopamine antagonist that sensitizes the GI tissues to the action of acetylcholine.

3. _____ are weak bases that can be ingested to neutralize the hydrochloric acid secreted by the stomach.

4. _____ drugs block muscarinic receptors, inhibit gastric acid secretion, and depress GI motility.

5. _____ (Carafate) is a complex of sulfated sucrose and aluminum hydroxide.

6. _____ (Cytotec) is an ester of prostaglandin E$_1$ and represents a new drug class for treating ulcers.

7./8. _____ and

_____ are the drugs of choice for treating motion sickness and vertigo.

9. _____ are used as antiemetic therapy for cancer chemotherapy.

10. _____, camphorated opium tincture, is used to treat diarrhea.

11. Bismuth _____ are effective in controlling traveler's diarrhea by binding the bacterial toxins.

12. An opioid used to control diarrhea, _____ _____ can be given orally or administered intramuscularly.

13. _____, the most effective nonspecific antidiarrheals, decrease the tone of the small and large intestines in a manner that slows the transit of material.

14. _____ is a synthetic disaccharide that is not hydrolyzed by intestinal enzymes and is not absorbed.

15. _____ (irritant) cathartics include cascara, danthron, senna, phenolphthalein, bisacodyl, castor oil, and glycerin.

FILL IN THE BLANK

16. How does one assess a patient with suspected ulcer disease?

_____

_____

_____

_____

_____

_____

Drugs to Improve Circulation

Hidden in each box on this page are five words or phrases — four related items or conditions, plus a fifth word that identifies what these four have in common. Each word or phrase is divided into five parts and concealed sequentially from left to right in consecutive columns. For example, one of the phrases in box #1 is CLAMMY SKIN, with the letters CL in the first column, AM in the second, MY in the third, SK in the fourth, and IN in the fifth. The category, SHOCK, of which the other four phrases are all symptoms, is similarly concealed in left-to-right fashion. Now see if you can find the three remaining symptoms. Then try the other boxes on your own. You may cross out squares as you solve, because each will be used only once. The term or phrase representing the overall category for each box has been done for you.

cl	po	o̶	ath	se
hy	pid	ten	pul	in
thr	h̶	my	sk	on
s̶	ea	bre	si	k̶
ra	am	dy	e̶	ing

1. clammy skin _____ _____

   shock _____ _____

   _____

cy	un	up	a̶t̶	te
fl	s̶o̶	ar	ela	ne
iso	cla	dip	ri	ine
v̶a̶	mo	nd	iz	o̶r̶s̶
ni	xs	d̶i̶l̶	i	ne

3. vasodilators _____ _____

   _____ _____

fa	lat	r̶o̶	lci	oo	a	ts
re	t̶h̶e̶	y	dbl	lp	o̶s̶	ion
col	tt	e	s̶e̶	po	lat	ow
a̶	duc	era	na	l̶e̶r̶	dfl	i̶s̶
a	ng	i	de	rcu	si	in

2. atherosclerosis _____ _____

   _____ _____

   _____

da	rn	rya	t̶a̶	tr	pa	m
v̶a̶	cc	lyr	h	p	i̶n̶	st
o	ona	a̶n̶	ge	rys	th	a̶
mo	t̶i̶	in	ra	n̶g̶	iso	sm
cor	i	u	rte	y	e	des

4. variant angina _____ _____

   _____ _____

   _____

CHAPTER 15

Antihypertensive Drugs

Below is the framework for a model for the stepped-care regimen for treatment of hypertension. Complete the model by writing *inside each step* the appropriate actions to be taken for each.

Stepped-Care Regimen for Hypertension

Step 4

Step 3

Step 2

Step 1

Nonpharmacologic recommendations:

Antihypertensive Drugs

Begin by filling in the four blank lines at the top, which identify the four categories of antihypertensive agents. Below each list a specific agent within each category. Finally, choose one drug for which to identify indications, side effects, and patient teaching strategies.

I. _____   II. _____   III. _____   IV. _____

e.g. _____   e.g. _____   e.g. _____   e.g. _____

Specific antihypertensive agent: _____

Indications: _____

Side effects: _____

_____

Teach patient: _____

_____

_____

_____

CHAPTER 16

Diuretics

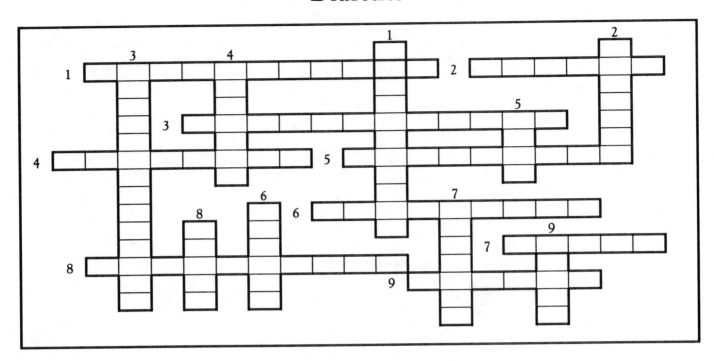

ACROSS

1. _____ is a balanced condition in which the body retains the salt and water required for proper function and eliminates the excess.
2. Chloride ion is primarily removed from tubular fluid in the ascending limb of _____ loop.
3. Two potassium-sparing diuretics should not be given _____.
4. Benzthiazide, cyclothiazide, and Diuril are all examples of _____ diuretics.
5. Carbonic anhydrase inhibitors have diuretic action because _____ accompanies the excreted bicarbonate.
6. While _____ ion is not the primary ion involved in the action of a diuretic drug, its excretion is nonetheless altered by some of these agents.
7. _____ vegetables are a good source of potassium.
8. _____ is the loop diuretic most likely to be included in hypertension therapy.
9. The ___ is the primary site for maintenance of water balance.

DOWN

1. The main buffer for the blood.
2. The functional unit of the kidney.
3. Many drugs enter tubular fluid by a mechanism called the _____ (3 words).
4. _____ diuretics are nonelectrolytes filtered by the glomerulus, but not significantly reabsorbed or metabolized.
5. Bumetanide inhibits the active reabsorption of chloride ions in the ascending _____ of Henle's loop.
6. Bumetanide is more _____ than other loop diuretics.
7. Potassium-_____ diuretics inhibit the pump mechanism that normally exchanges potassium for sodium in the distal convoluted tubule.
8. Fluid entering the proximal convoluted tubule has the same sodium ion content as _____.
9. Conditions responding to diuretics include pulmonary, renal, and brain _____.

CHAPTER 17

Fluids and Electrolytes

BUBBLES

The answer to each of the clues in this puzzle is a five-letter word related to fluids and electrolytes. Enter each word into the grid by placing its first letter in the center of the correspondingly numbered bubble, and the remaining letters in the four outer spaces, proceeding counterclockwise. It's up to you to determine where the outer four letters begin in each bubble. Good luck!

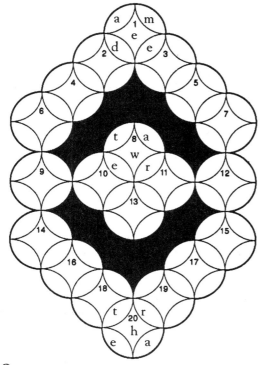

CLUES

1. When assessing a patient's need for fluids and electrolytes observe for _____, especially in dependent areas; check skin turgor; auscultate breath and heart sounds; monitor vital signs, weight, and intake and output.
2. Patients unable to take oral _____ and fluids require maintenance with IV nutrients.
3. It is important to remember to _____ all IV fluids and medications carefully, monitor their rate of flow and their effects, and record carefully.
4. _____ acids are used in TPN to prevent negative nitrogen balance and breakdown of protein in the body.
5. Ringer's solution is used to replace fluid, sodium, and other electrolytes; they are appropriate to replace volume if _____ function is not seriously compromised.

6. Dextrose in water may be used to _____ fluid from the interstitial space into the plasma.
7. Metabolic acidosis arises when excess acid is produced, as in diabetic acidosis, lactic acidosis, starvation, or certain _____ of poisoning.
8. Osmosis is the movement of _____ across a semipermeable membrane.
9. Intracellular fluid comprises the water inside _____ and its dissolved solute.
10. Dextran and hetastarch are complex carbohydrate molecules too _____ to pass out of the capillaries or vascular walls thereby acting as plasma expanders.
11. Metabolic alkalosis can _____ when excess hydrogen ions are lost, as in prolonged vomiting or nasogastric suctioning.
12. Administer IV fat emulsions during TPN to prevent _____ acid deficiency.
13. When assessing a patient's fluid and electrolyte status observe for _____ of nutritional deficiency, remembering that weight and intake measures alone are poor indicators.
14. _____ and electrolyte therapy is effective if desired goals have been achieved without harmful consequences to the patient.
15. If fluid loss is excessive and uncompensated, the patient may enter hypovolemic _____, in which the blood volume becomes so depleted that organ perfusion is compromised.
16. Symptoms of hypovolemic shock include lowered blood pressure, increased heart rate, _____ respiration, restlessness, pale and clammy skin, and decreased urine output.
17. Hypernatremia (excessive sodium ion concentration in plasma) arises when a patient _____ water and retains salt.
18. Ringer's solution is appropriate replacement therapy for patients who have lost fluid and electrolytes through the alimentary _____ for burn patients, for postoperative patients, and for patients with dehydration and sodium depletion.
19. Oncotic pressure is balanced by hydrostatic pressure generated by the _____ of contraction of the heart.
20. Hyperkalemia (excessive potassium ion concentration in the plasma) can be life threatening because _____ function may be impaired.

Cardiac Glycosides and Other Drugs for Congestive Heart Failure

TRUE OR FALSE

_____ 1. Automaticity is the ability of certain heart cells to depolarize spontaneously to initiate a beat (contraction of the whole heart).

_____ 2. Normally, a heartbeat is initiated in the atrioventricular (AV) node.

_____ 3. Any of the conductive fibers of the heart are capable of spontaneously depolarizing and initiating beats and do so in certain types of heart disease.

_____ 4. The heart is formed of muscle similar in many respects to skeletal muscle in that many of the fibers conduct as well as contract.

_____ 5. The peak efficiency of the heart is 175 to 200 beats/min. Faster rates result in incomplete filling of the ventricles and reduce the overall efficiency of the pump.

_____ 6. The Frank-Starling law states that the force of muscular contraction is directly related to the stretch of the muscle; the more a muscle is stretched, within mechanical limits, the stronger its subsequent contraction.

_____ 7. Hypertrophy of the myocardium may occur if the heart is subjected to chronic demands for increased output and may be a normal response to chronic stress.

_____ 8. In congestive heart failure, the blood pools in the veins, producing increased venous pressure; as excessive venous pressure stretches cardiac muscle fibers beyond their limit, the strength of contraction falls further.

_____ 9. The symptoms of congestive heart failure may be reduced by decreasing cardiac output.

_____ 10. Biochemically, cardiac glycosides work because they inhibit Na+, K+, -ATPase and promote accumulation within the heart cells of the calcium necessary for contraction.

_____ 11. Because of the long half-life of cardiac glycosides, administration is often initiated with a loading dose.

_____ 12. Digitoxin is usually given intramuscularly in a dose to produce and maintain the therapeutic level in plasma of 14 to 26 ng/ml.

_____ 13. Digoxin differs from digitoxin with its shorter half life and is less highly bound to plasma protein.

_____ 14. Deslanoside is the cardiac glycoside of choice when considering long-term therapy for CHF.

_____ 15. Dobutamime, dopamine, and amrinone are adrenergic receptors in the heart increasing cardiac contractility by increasing cyclic adenosine monophosphate (cAMP) in heart muscle.

_____ 16. Diuretics control pulmonary edema that accompanies severe congestive heart failure.

_____ 17. The major consideration limiting use of diuretics in CHF is the risk of causing electrolyte or fluid imbalances.

_____ 18. Vasodilators as a class have limited usefulness.

_____ 19. Captopril and enalapril are angiotensin-converting enzyme (ACE) inhibitors.

_____ 20. There are no special considerations to take into account when administering cardiac glycosides to the elderly.

MATCHING

_____ 1. Depolarization

_____ 2. Excitability

_____ 3. Action potential

_____ 4. Conduction velocity

_____ 5. Dromotropic

_____ 6. Bradycardia

_____ 7. Tachycardia

_____ 8. Chronotropic

_____ 9. Contractility

_____ 10. Inotropic

a. factors affecting conduction velocity

b. measure of the ease with which a cell may be stimulated to depolarize

c. slow heart rate

d. changes in heart rate

e. measured as strength of muscular contraction of the heart

f. factors affecting strength of cardiac contraction

g. fast heart rate

h. rate at which an electrical impulse passes through the AV node

i. Process by which cells become less negatively charged than extracellular fluid

j. burst of electrical activity in a cell

Drugs To Control Cardiac Arrythmias

Hidden in each box on this page are five words related to cardiac arrhythmias. Solve each of the clues below the boxes, writing the correct word on each blank. If your answer is correct you will find it hidden in the corresponding box, its parts concealed sequentially from left to right in consecutive columns. For example, one of the words in box #1 is PACING, with the letter P in the first column, A in the second, C in the third, I in the fourth, N in the fifth, and G in the sixth.

G	A	O	I	L	E
P	U	O	C	N	S
M	R	C	U	K	S
B	L	S	I	P	N
A	C	T	C	O	G

1._____ 2._____

3._____ 4._____

5._____

1. Arrhythmias occur because of disorders in the _____ of the heartbeat or in conducting the impulse to beat through heart tissues.
2. Ectopic foci are _____ of cells in the atria or the ventricles that spontaneously beat independently of the SA node.
3. If an area of heart _____ becomes ischemic or damaged, it may not only fail to contract, but it may also fail to properly conduct an action potential.
4. Moricizine _____ sodium channels, as well as potent local anesthetic activity and membrane-stabilizing activity.
5. Quinidine and procainamide have virtually identical mechanisms of _____.

A	O	T	A	E
T	L	X	I	L
A	O	R	I	R
L	T	C	E	C
A	M	I	D	A

6._____ 7._____

8._____ 9._____

10._____

6. The primary difference between quinidine and procainamide is in the _____ effects produced.
7. Class I-B antiarrhythmic drugs have much less effect on _____ than the class I-A drugs.
8. Lidocaine is a _____ anesthetic that alters sodium ion conduction in heart cells.
9. Phenytoin, a drug used as an anticonvulsant, may _____ cardiac function by CNS effects.
10. Tocainide, like lidocaine, is an _____-type of local anesthetic.

M	A	G	O	L
R	C	C	I	R
O	R	P	U	T
T	A	N	A	D
V	I	E	A	R

11._____ 12._____

13._____ 14._____

15._____

11. Paroxysmal supraventricular tachycardia is a _____ heart rate produced by sudden overactivity in the atria.
12. Sinus bradycardia is usually of _____ importance and not treated.
13. Premature ventricular contractions _____ when the ventricles beat in response to both the SA node and an abnormal pacemaker.
14. Atropine, most often used as a blocker of muscarinic cholinergic receptors, can also _____ certain arrhythmias.
15. Digitalis can strengthen contraction of the heart muscle and it also increases _____ tone at the AV node.

Agents Affecting Blood Coagulation

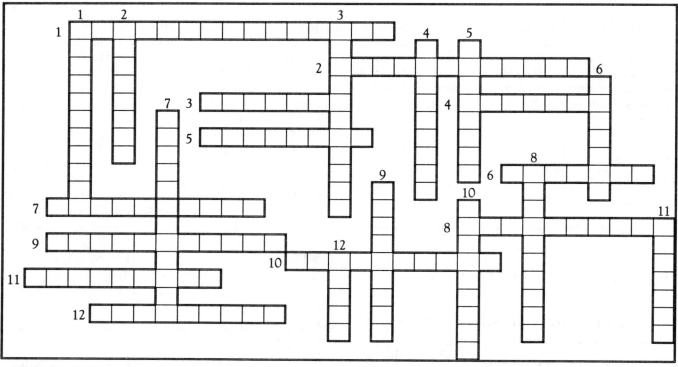

ACROSS

1. This process prevents clot formation; it does not dissolve existing clots.
2. _____ (Persantine) combines with warfarin for patients with artificial heart valves.
3. _____ is an anticoagulant that can either be administered to the patient or added to a storage container.
4. A dislodged thrombus in the arterial or venous system.
5. The most widely used coumarin.
6. _____ is a cofactor for each of the steps through the activation of prothrombin.
7. The major side effect of heparin.
8. Systemic _____ drugs include epsilon, aminocaproic acid (Amicar), tranexamic acid (Cyklokapron), and vitamin K.
9. _____ (Ticlid) inhibits platelet aggregation irreversibly and may be effective in preventing strokes and MI.
10. _____ is an inherited disorder in which there is a deficiency of one of the factors necessary for coagulation of the blood.
11. Desmopressin is a synthetic analogue of the _____ hormone, vasopressin.
12. Effective in treating coronary thrombosis, streptokinase (_____) is isolated from group C beta-hemolytic streptococci; it is one tenth the cost of alteplase treatment.

DOWN

1. _____ (Miradon) is the only indandione approved for use in the U.S. and Canada.
2. Another name for blood clot
3. Although drug interactions are uncommon with _____ they cause frequent side effects including rash, bone marrow depression, hepatitis, and renal damage.
4. _____ (Abbokinase) is isolated from human urine; it is an enzyme that cleaves plasminogen to plasmin.
5. Local absorbable hemostatics provide a surface that promotes platelet _____ and blood clotting.
6. The most widely studied and used antiplatelet drug.
7. Anisoylated Plasminogen-Streptokinase Activator Complex
8. Gelatin sponge, gelatin film, oxidized cellulose, microfibrillar collagen hemostat, and thrombin comprise the local _____ hemostatics.
9. _____ (Activase; TPA) is produced for pharmacologic use by recombinant DNA technology
10. Hemophilia B or _____ disease is an inherited X-linked recessive disorder characterized by a deficiency of factor IX.
11. Hemophilia A, or _____ hemophilia is a deficiency of factor VIII, which is important in the activation of factor X.
12. Hemophilia A is inherited as an X-linked recessive disorder and seen almost exclusively in _____.

Drugs to Lower Blood Lipid Levels

TOSSED-WORD PUZZLE

Unscramble the terms below and write them in the blanks below each to reveal words associated with blood lipid levels; then define the term. Next, unscramble the marked letters to fill in the blank under the clue.

1. I P D S L I

□ _ _ □ _ _

2. A N N I C I

_ _ □ _ _ □

3. R U L A C V S A

□ _ □ _ _ _ □ _

4. T O X R I T H Y R O N E X D E

_ _ _ □ _ □ □ _ _ _ _ _ _ _

CLUE: It may be "love" but not to low-density lipoproteins!

_ _ _ _ _ _ _ _ _ _ _

COMPLETE THE SENTENCES

5. _____ is the gradual blocking of arteries by a buildup of plaque.

6. Lipids are bound to special proteins to form soluble

_____ .

7. Name the four major classes of lipoproteins:

_____ ,

_____ ,

_____ , and

_____ .

8. _____ and _____ are largely composed of triglycerides and transport triglycerides to tissues for metabolic use or storage.

9. _____ and _____ transport cholesterol.

10. _____ is an abnormal concentration of one or more of the four lipoproteins.

MATCHING

___1. Cholestyramine

___2. Clofibrate

___3. Gemfibrozil

___4. Lovastatin

___5. Aluminum nicotinate

___6. Dextrothyroxine

___7. Probucol

___8. Conjugated estrogens

___9. Androgens

___10. Neomycin

A. Chemically related to clofibrate. Interferes with the transfer of fatty acids from adipose tissue to the liver and with hepatic production of VLDL.
B. Resin with a sandlike texture that stays in the intestine and binds bile acids.
C. B vitamin, at many times the minimum daily requirement useful in treating types II, III, IV, and V hyperlipidemias.
D. Inactive stereo-isomer of the hormone thyroxine.
E. It decreases plasma LDL and cholesterol, potentially useful in treating type II hyperlipidemia.
F. May reduce elevated plasma triglyceride concentrations in males only.
G. Used as lipid-lowering agents because premenopausal women have a low incidence of MI.
H. An antibiotic that is not well absorbed—prevents cholesterol adsorption in the intestine, thereby promoting bile acid secretion.
I. Reduces plasma concentration of triglycerides by activating the enzyme lipoprotein lipase and inhibiting the release of VLDL by the liver. Produces few side effects.
J. Reduces plasma concentration of triglycerides by activating the enzyme lipoprotein lipase and inhibiting the release of VLDL by the liver. Produces few side effects.

Drugs to Treat Anemia

In the puzzles below, you are to fit the letters in each column into the boxes directly above them in order to form words. The letters may or may not go into the boxes in the same order in which they are given. It is up to you to decide which letter goes into which box above it. Once a letter is used, it cannot be used again. A ♦ indicates the end of a word. When a diagram has been filled in, it will be your clue for solving the puzzle.

Puzzle 1

		♦		O	D	Y		♦				♦				♦	M	E	C					♦
	♦	R	E					♦	E	X						♦			O	N	;		♦	
M	U		♦				K	E	♦				♦						♦	I	R			
	E	R				♦				L	E	D	:	♦	♦	♦	♦	♦	♦	♦	♦	♦	♦	
~~M~~	V	~~E~~	~~R~~	L	I	A	T	A	C	A	S	~~L~~	~~E~~	~~D~~	S	C	I	R	S	A	N	~~I~~	~~R~~	M	N
O	O	~~C~~	~~R~~	E	M	N	V	E	H	A	~~X~~	C	N	S		~~M~~	A	~~C~~	H	~~N~~		I	T	O	O
T	H	E	H	B	~~O~~	~~D~~	D		~~K~~	~~L~~	L	C	E	N			~~L~~	U	~~O~~	E				S	O
T	~~U~~			O	O	~~Y~~			~~L~~			A	O												

1. _____ (1 word)

Puzzle 2

R	E	D	♦					♦	C	E				♦	R	E	L					D	♦	♦	♦
			♦				♦			G	E	♦				♦		M					♦	♦	
	A	U	S		♦			♦		D	E			C		E	N			Y	♦		♦		
	♦			♦	S	Y	N						♦		♦	♦	♦	♦	♦	♦	♦	♦	♦		
~~R~~	F	A	T	B	~~S~~	R	~~Y~~	F	T	~~E~~	H	S	I	S	~~E~~	I	S	~~C~~	A	~~N~~	C	U	R	E	
O	~~E~~	~~D~~	~~A~~	N	A	O	O	D	L	A	T	E	~~E~~	S	A	N	F	I	I	~~M~~	S	A	T	~~Y~~	
T	E	C	D	~~U~~	L	E	E	O	~~N~~	~~C~~	H	~~G~~	E		~~D~~	~~R~~	~~L~~	E	I	M	E	~~D~~			
B	~~H~~			~~A~~				R	L	L				D											

2. _____ (3 words)

Puzzle 3

S	P			I	A		♦						G	♦	P	R	O					♦
R		Q					♦	F			♦	V	I					♦	B	1	2	
T	R					♦	I		T		♦				♦	♦	♦	♦	♦	♦	♦	
		E		I	N	A		♦	C			S		♦	♦	♦	♦	♦	♦	♦	♦	
~~T~~	~~R~~	~~Q~~	N	I	T	O	~~N~~	~~A~~	L	O	~~C~~	~~T~~	~~Y~~	L	~~S~~	H	~~R~~	I	N	E	I	~~1~~	~~2~~
~~R~~	E	A	~~E~~	S	~~A~~	L	R	T	I	~~1~~	N	E	L	~~1~~	T	A	E	~~O~~	T		~~B~~	N
I	N	T	C	~~1~~	P	~~1~~	D	B	~~F~~	N	R	I	O	~~C~~	T	~~P~~	M					
~~S~~	~~P~~	E	U	S	R	E					D		N									

3. _____ (2 words)

CHAPTER 23
Drugs for Pain and Inflammation

TRUE OR FALSE

_____ 1. An analgesic-antipyretic drug relieves pain but doesn't reduce fever.

_____ 2. Aspirin and acetaminophen are the major analgesic-antipyretic drugs.

_____ 3. Nonnarcotic analgesics inhibit cyclooxygenase.

_____ 4. The mechanism of action for the nonnarcotic analgesics is similar to that of the narcotic analgesics.

_____ 5. The thermostat of the body is an area of the preoptic anterior hypothalamus.

_____ 6. The over-the-counter salicylates not only produce analgesia and antipyresis, they rarely cause side effects or produce drug interactions.

_____ 7. Acetaminophen is preferred to aspirin in treating fever in childhood because it has not been implicated in the development of Reye's syndrome as has aspirin.

_____ 8. Aspirin is an alternative to acetaminophen because it does not cause gastric irritation or alter platelet binding and bleeding times as does acetaminophen.

_____ 9. At high doses (3 to 6 gm/day) aspirin treats the inflammation of rheumatoid arthritis and acts as a prototype for the NSAIDs.

_____ 10. Aspirin can be used as a prophylactic agent to prevent myocardial infarction and strokes because it inhibits blood clotting.

MULTIPLE CHOICE
Circle the correct answer.

11. Patients allergic to aspirin show cross-sensitivity to:
A. apples, oranges, and bananas   D. diclofenac
B. iodide-containing substances   E. all of the above.
C. tartrazine

12. The following drugs have been implicated in Reye's syndrome.
A. acetaminophen   D. diclofenac
B. ibuprofen   E. all of the above
C. aspirin

13. A derivative of salicylic acid with a long duration of action, _____ is a compound taken orally that relieves the symptoms of rheumatoid arthritis and osteoarthritis with fewer side effects than aspirin.
A. diflunisal   C. thiosalicylate
B. Olsalazine   D. all of the above

14. In treating rheumatoid arthritis, drugs that may alter the progression of joint erosion include:
A. gold therapy   D. immunosuppressive drugs
B. hydroxychloroquine E. all of the above
C. penicillamine

MATCHING

___15. Methotrexate

___16. Glucocorticoids

___17. Auranofin

___18. Aurothioglucose

___19. Azathioprine

___20. Ketorolac tromethamine

___21. Ibuprofen

___22. Mefenamic acid

___23. Piroxicam

A. A gold compound that can be taken orally
B. NSAID derived from propionic acid, as are fenoprofen, floctafenine, flurbiprofen and naproxen.
C. New NSAID principally used as analgesic with equivalent potency to morphine
D. Immunosuppressive agent used to suppress rejection in organ transplantation. Manages severe active arthritis unresponsive to conventional medications.
E. Injectable gold salts
F. Folic acid antagonist used to treat cancer and psoriasis.
G. Dramatically relieves inflammation and accompanying pain of arthritis. Does not alter course of disease.
H. NSAID prescribed principally for rheumatoid arthritis and osteoarthritis. Well absorbed with long half life, making once-a-day dosing adequate.
I. An antimalarial drug used as an alternative to gold therapy in treatment of arthritis.

Antihistamines

HIDDEN AGENDA

Terms relating to the antihistamines are hidden in the grid below. They may appear vertically, horizontally, diagonally, left-to-right, or right-to-left. First solve the clues below then locate each term in the grid by either highlighting or circling it.

H	I	S	T	A	M	I	N	E	A	B	D	I	S	A	C	H
A	C	C	O	N	L	N	I	M	R	J	P	R	O	R	O	A
N	I	N	O	G	Q	U	I	L	X	D	O	U	R	T	N	Y
T	G	R	H	I	N	I	T	I	S	T	C	Z	U	E	T	F
I	R	M	O	O	N	I	F	C	P	L	R	M	J	R	R	E
H	E	L	J	E	M	S	T	E	I	N	O	R	C	I	A	V
I	N	F	M	D	A	L	C	O	H	O	L	T	S	O	I	E
S	I	R	J	E	M	E	N	I	E	I	M	U	R	L	N	R
T	L	Q	I	M	R	J	E	M	E	N	I	E	I	E	D	C
A	O	A	N	A	P	H	Y	L	A	X	I	S	T	S	I	O
M	H	S	T	L	U	R	T	I	C	A	R	I	A	Z	C	C
I	C	T	B	A	R	Y	Z	R	S	P	N	L	M	T	A	D
N	I	H	N	B	P	G	R	C	O	L	D	S	N	I	T	S
E	T	M	M	N	U	C	I	S	N	E	M	C	S	R	E	C
R	N	A	J	B	R	O	N	C	H	I	A	L	W	R	D	T
F	A	I	D	R	A	C	Y	H	C	A	T	W	R	T	O	I
S	T	I	M	U	L	A	T	I	O	N	N	C	S	M	A	I

1. _____ is a naturally-occurring amine that is formed from the amino acid histidine.

2. Swelling caused by plasma leakage and blood vessel didation in the skin or mucous membranes is _____ _____.

3. _____ is indicated by itching and tingling sensation followed by profound hypotension leading to shock.

4. _____ is the spasm of the bronchial smooth muscle.

5. What red spots on the skin are caused by the leakage of blood from small vessels?_____

6. _____ is an inflammation of the nasal mucous membranes that allows fluid to escape.

7. The definition of _____ is hives, which are large wheals caused by leakage of plasma and are accompanied by severe itching.

Two actions of histamine are prominent in explaining allergic responses:

8. Histamine is a potent dilator of _____ and renders capillaries more permeable so that fluid and protein are lost into the extravascular space.

9. Histamine also stimulates the contraction of smooth muscle, particularly _____ smooth muscle.

10. There are two types of histamine _____ _____: H-1 receptors, acting on blood vessels and bronchioles, and the H-2 receptors, acting mainly on the GI tract.

11. The term _____ refers to drugs that specifically block the H-1 receptors.

12. The antihistamines have secondary properties—among them their _____ or atropine-like action.

13. Some of the side effects of the antihistamines are inhibition of secretion, blurred vision, urinary retention, fast heart rate (_____) and constipation.

14. Antihistamine overdose can cause CNS depression or _____, the latter being more common in children.

15. Drug interaction associated with antihistamines are the additive depression of the CNS when taken with _____, hypnotics, sedatives, or narcotic analgesics.

16. Antihistamines are _____ for nursing mothers because the drugs are secreted in milk.

17. _____ is most successfully treated when the antihistamine therapy is begun while the pollen count is still low.

18. Although present in many cold remedies, antihistamines do not prevent or treat _____ effectively.

CHAPTER 25

Bronchodilators and Other Drugs to Treat Asthma

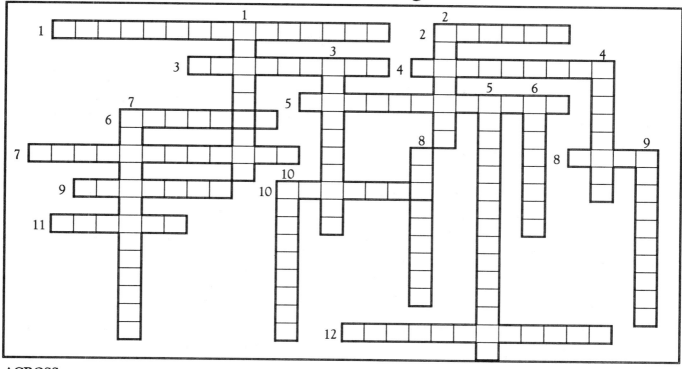

ACROSS

1. Drugs that dilate the bronchioles are called _____.
2. _____ is a disease of reversible obstruction of the bronchioles.
3. Asthma is classified as _____ if an allergic response is the primary stimulus for bronchial constriction.
4. _____ such as noxious gases can stimulate guanyl cyclase, the enzyme that triggers intrinsic asthma.
5. Cromolyn sodium is a valuable _____ in treatment of mild asthma since it prevents the mast cells from degranulating to start an asthma attack.
6. Infants born at less than 37 weeks gestation are at risk for respiratory distress syndrome, also called _____ membrane disease.
7. _____, a long-acting oral bronchodilator, is widely used as daily therapy for moderate to severe asthma.
8. _____ asthma is managed with a beta-adrenergic inhalant bronchodilator.
9. Because the newer beta-adrenergic bronchodilators are relatively selective, these drugs are less likely to cause unwanted _____ effects.
10. Lung damage in COPD results from the destruction of _____, a major structural protein of the lung.
11. Cyclic AMP activates intracellular pathways, resulting in relaxation of smooth _____, inhibition of mast cell degranulation, and stimulation of the ciliary apparatus.

12. Ephedrine, epinephrine and isoproterenol are not selective for the beta-2 adrenergic receptor and have a wide range of side effects resulting from their _____ action.

DOWN

1. Asthma is classified as _____ if a cause cannot be identified.
2. Chronic obstructive pulmonary disease (COPD) describes the conditions in which there is limited _____.
3. _____ is a lipoprotein material coating the air sacs in mature lungs, lowering surface tension and allowing ready inflation of the lungs.
4. Inhaled _____ are preferred over theophylline as daily therapy for moderate to severe asthma because there are fewer side effects.
5. Antihistamines can be administered to prevent mild episodes, but they are _____ in patients with severe asthma.
6. There is _____ innervation of the bronchioles by the sympathetic nervous system, since sympathetic nerve terminals in pulmonary blood vessels release norepinephrine that act on the beta-2 receptors in the bronchioles.
7. Drug therapy for asthma aims to prevent bronchospasm and to control _____ of the bronchioles.
8. Theophylline and related drugs are known as _____.
9. _____ is related to theophylline but is less potent and shorter acting.
10. Chronic bronchitis and _____ are referred to as chronic obstructive pulmonary disease.

CHAPTER 26

Drugs to Control Bronchial Secretions

MATCHING

___1. Phenylephrine   ___9. Antitussive

___2. Phenylpropanolamine   ___10. Codeine

___3. Propylhexedrine   ___11. Hydrocodone

___4. Imidazolines   ___12. Dextromethorphan

___5. Naphazoline   ___13. Chlorphedianol

___6. Oxymetazoline   ___14. Mucolytics

___7. Expectorant   ___15. Acetylcysteine

___8. Guaifenesin

A. Group of four chemically related nasal decongestants which stimulate the alpha-adrenergic receptors to produce vasoconstriction.

B. Volatile drug that stimulates alpha receptors. Causes little stimulation of the CNS; therefore safer than other nasal decongestants.

C. Relatively long-lasting decongestant that has not been implicated in as many severe systemic effects as naphazoline.

D. Drugs that act as a cough suppressant—from the Latin word meaning cough.

E. Opiate with a greater potential for producing drug dependence than codeine.

F. Group of drugs that break up viscous mucus so that it can be coughed up or drained.

G. A sulfhydryl compound that can break disulfide bonds. Administered by nebulizer through a face mask, mouthpiece or tracheostomy.

H. Decongestant used mainly in oral combination cold remedies. An alpha-adrenergic agonist that acts indirectly, releasing norepinephrine from nerve terminals.

I. An effective nasal decongestant, but can produce severe rebound congestion.

J. A decongestant with potent alpha-adrenergic agonist effects that is administered orally or topically.

K. Most widely used antitussive in OTC cough mixtures.

L. Centrally-acting antitussive with local anesthetic and anticholinergic action.

M. Widely used expectorant for which there is some evidence of efficacy.

N. Increases the output of respiratory tract fluid to coat trachea and bronchi; has not been proven effective.

O. A good antitussive, but an opiate and capable of producing drug dependence.

TRUE OR FALSE

_____ 16. Nasal congestion results when the blood vessels in the nasal passage become dilated as a result of infection, inflammation, allergy, or emotional upset.

_____ 17. Topical nasal decongestants are effective, cause few side effects, and are safe to use for extended periods of time.

_____ 18. Patients with hyperthyroidism, diabetes mellitus, and hypertension are vulnerable to the sympathomimetic side effects of nasal decongestants and should avoid them.

_____ 19. The mucociliary escalator provides a cleansing mechanism for the lungs, since any foreign particle or bacteria are trapped in a viscous layer and eliminated.

_____ 20. A cough is a protective reflex initiated by irritation in the airway. As long as material is being brought up by the cough it is beneficial.

26

CHAPTER 27

Basic Function of the Immune System

BUBBLES

The answer to each of the clues in this puzzle is a five-letter word related to the function of the immune system. Enter each word into the grid by placing its first letter in the center of the correspondingly numbered bubble, and the remaining letters in the four outer spaces, proceeding clockwise. It's up to you to determine where the outer four letters begin in each bubble. Good luck!

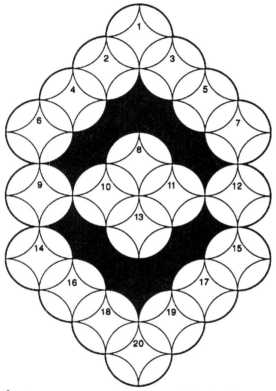

1. Any foreign _____ capable of inducing an immune response is termed an antigen.
2. Heavy _____ disease is characterized by the appearance of large amounts of protein in the serum and urine resembling the Fc portion of the immunoglobulin molecule.
3. Phagocytosis is ingestion and destruction of foreign particles such as bacteria by individual _____ of the immune system.
4. Macrophages may be fixed within the tissues, where they may persist for _____; some however, recirculate through secondary lymphoid organs.
5. An eosinophil participates in allergic reaction and _____ parasites.
6. Lympho-_____ are subdivided in thymus-derived or T cells and the bone-marrow-derived or B cells.

7. Patients with T cell disorders are extremely susceptible to fungal, _____, and protozoal infections.
8. Secondary immunodeficiencies _____ as complications of other diseases.
9. _____ deficiencies affect not only cell-mediated immune responses but also synthesis of antibodies, since they are necessary for most antibody responses.
10. Infants with severe combined immunodeficiencies can be _____ by bone marrow transplantation.
11. Cytotoxic T cells reject grafts and destroy _____ infected cells.
12. The complement system is a system of enzymes found in _____.
13. A _____ patch is a cluster of lymphocytes spread throughout the lining of the intestinal wall, tonsils, and appendix.
14. The spleen, lymph _____ and Peyer's patches are the secondary lympohid organs.
15. Excess immunoglobulin _____ to increased viscosity of serum, which leads to decreased blood flow, thrombosis, disorders of the CNS, and bleeding.
16. Major functions of the complement system include opsonization of antigenic particles which cause damage to the membrane of pathogens that often result in _____ of the pathogen, and mediating inflammatory responses.
17. The _____ of helper cells to cytotoxic cells normally ranges from 1.2:2 to 2:1.
18. PMNs are the predominant phagocytes within the circulation. They are usually the _____ cells to arrive at the site of an infection.
19. Acquired immunity is not present at _____ but develops as the individual grows and matures.
20. The immune system is comprised of six _____ blood cell types: lymphocytes, monocytes and macrophages, polymorphonuclear leukocytes, basophils, mast cells, and eosinophils.

Immunomodulators

Hidden in each box on this page are five words related to immunomodulators. Each word is divided into parts and concealed sequentially from left to right in consecutive columns. For example, one of the words in box #1 is IMMUNE, with the letter I in the first column, M in the second, M in the third, U in the fourth, N in the fifth, and E in the sixth. Identify, on the blanks below, each word hidden in the accompanying box. Cross out squares as you find each word, because each will be used only once.

I	C	F	U	N	E
A	M	L	I	V	T
B	I	T	A	N	T
K	N	M	L	S	D
I	R	E	A	E	E

1. IMMUNE   4. _____

2. _____   5. _____

3. _____

1. Immunostimulants enhance or stimulate the _____ system.
2. Vaccines usually contain _____ or attenuated bacteria or viruses, but protection can also be conferred with immunogenic proteins or toxoids from the pathogen.
3. _____ immunity usually persists for years.
4. A newborn _____ does not have a fully functional immune system; but human milk does contain factors that aid the newborn response against infectious agents.
5. Some of the factors in _____ milk enhance the growth of beneficial intestinal flora, and others nonspecifically inhibit the growth of harmful microorganisms.

W	E	E	K	O
B	E	T	U	M
S	O	G	I	N
P	E	R	I	S
F	E	L	U	S

6. _____   9. _____

7. _____   10. _____

8. _____

6. Infant immunizations can _____ at 2 months of age when the baby can mount an effective immune response of its own.
7. Live virus vaccines are contraindicated in pregnant women since they can damage the _____.

8. Passive immunity, which lasts only _____, involves administration of preformed substances such as immune serum or antibodies that can immediately combat the foreign agent to which they are directed.
9. Vaccines are administered by either IM or subcutaneous injection. The exceptions are the smallpox vaccine, which is given intradermally and the oral vaccine for

_____.
10. An immune _____, especially those using nonhuman proteins, can cause anaphylaxis in patients with a history of hypersensitivity reactions to immune globulin injections.

S	A	N	N	C	R
M	I	R	C	A	W
A	I	G	R	E	T
D	C	T	E	V	L
C	A	R	I	O	E

11. _____   14. _____

12. _____   15. _____

13. _____

11. _____ acquired immunity involves administration of substances such as vaccines that stimulate the immune system to respond against foreign material.
12. New forms of therapy to treat _____ are the interferons and interleukins; the interferons also treat certain viral infections.
13. Interferon does not exhibit _____ antiviral action but acts indirectly within virus susceptible cells to mediate its antiviral effects.
14. Interferon binds to specific cell surface receptors, resulting in _____ transduction through the membrane and ultimately protein synthesis.
15. Colony stimulating factors induce the production of granulocytes in vivo, especially PMN; they are good candidates as adjuncts to cancer chemotherapy and bone _____ transplantation.

CHAPTER 29

Antiinfective and Chemotherapeutic Agents

TRUE OR FALSE

_____ 1. When Anton Van Leeuwenhoek discovered the microbial world in 1676 the impact of the discovery was immediately lauded.

_____ 2. Eucaryotic cells have genetic material that exists free within the cell protoplasm, whereas procaryotic cells have membrane-bound nuclei that contain the genetic material.

_____ 3. The poisoning of a disease-causing organism by means of an agent that has no effect on the person in whom the disease exists is known as selective toxicity.

_____ 4. The ratio of the dose of a certain drug that kills 50% of the animals tested is the therapeutic index.

_____ 5. Antibiotics act on microorganisms in one way: they inhibit cell wall formation.

_____ 6. It is misleading to classify a drug as exclusively bactericidal or bacteriostatic.

_____ 7. Antimicrobial spectrum is the type of microorganisms against which a particular drug is effective.

_____ 8. At one time all microorganisms were sensitive to antibiotics, now certain strains have become resistant.

_____ 9. Small circular pieces of DNA found separate from the chromosome in bacteria are called plasmids.

_____ 10. The precise mechanism of action by which a microorganism achieves resistance to an antibiotic may be divided in three categories.

SHORT ANSWERS

11. Before antibiotic therapy can begin what is the first step that needs to be taken?

_____

_____

_____

_____

12. What are some factors that influence the effectiveness of antibiotic therapy?

_____

_____

_____

_____

13. What is the most common misconception about antibiotics?

_____

_____

_____

_____

14. Why is it important to stress to patients not to discontinue therapy early?

_____

_____

_____

_____

15. What are some of the diseases caused by gram-negative bacteria?

_____

_____

_____

_____

_____

_____

_____

_____

Penicillins, Cephalosporins, and Related Drugs

DEFINITION PUZZLES

In the puzzles below, you are to fit the letters in each column into the boxes directly above them in order to form words. The letters may ar may not go into the boxes in the same order in which they are given. It is up to you to decide which letter goes into which box above it. Once a letter is used, cross it off the bottom half of the diagram and do not use it again. A black diamond indicates the end of a word. When the diagrams have been filled in, you will be able to answer the question the puzzle poses.

Puzzle 1

	E	◆	C	E	P	H				I		S	◆			
D	I	V			◆		N	T	◆	T		E		◆	◆	◆	◆
S	U	G			S	◆		N			◆		:	◆	◆	◆
~~S~~	~~I~~	~~V~~	~~G~~	~~C~~	O	U	~~H~~	~~S~~	~~N~~	~~T~~	~~N~~	O	~~T~~	~~H~~	~~R~~	~~E~~	~~E~~		A	R	E
~~D~~	~~U~~	~~E~~	I	D	~~E~~	~~P~~	P	I	L	O	O	P	O	R	~~I~~	A	~~S~~
T	H	B		R	E	D		A	K	S		W	N		N	S

ANSWER: _____

Puzzle 2

A	T	T	E	M			◆		◆		M	P	R		V		◆			◆	◆	◆	◆	◆	◆
			◆		B							◆			◆	P	E	N	I						
G	◆		E			◆		O	◆	D	E	V		O		M		◆		:	◆	◆	◆	◆
~~G~~	R	L	~~E~~	~~M~~	A	T	~~O~~	O	R	~~E~~	~~V~~	E	L	~~O~~	P	~~M~~	F	N	T	~~E~~	O	F	C	I	L	L	I	N
O	~~T~~	A	~~E~~	D	P	~~B~~	S		~~D~~	O	T	I	O	N	~~R~~	O	E	E	~~P~~	T	~~N~~	~~I~~
~~A~~		~~T~~	L		T	S		T	P		I	~~M~~	~~P~~		O	~~V~~			H	E

ANSWER: _____

Puzzle 3

W	H	Y	◆		◆	D	O	C			◆	P	E		F				◆	◆	◆
S	K		N	◆		E	S		◆	B		F	O		◆	◆	◆	◆	◆	◆	◆
									◆											
~~S~~	D	M	~~N~~	N	I	S	T	T	R	I	~~B~~	G	~~F~~	P	E	N	I	C	I	L	M	I	N	S
A	~~K~~	I	I	D	O	~~E~~	~~S~~	~~O~~	S	T	O	E	S	~~O~~	R	~~F~~	O	R	L
~~W~~	~~H~~	~~Y~~			T		~~D~~	E	~~C~~		N	R		~~P~~	E

ANSWER: _____

Puzzle 4

P	E	N	I					◆			D	◆	C	E	P		A									◆
	◆	N	O		◆	D				O	Y	◆						G	◆	◆	◆	◆	◆	◆	◆	◆
B	A	C				◆	C			◆	W	A		◆			◆									
	H		◆	F	O			A			O	N	◆		F	◆	W		◆	◆	◆	◆	◆	◆	◆	◆
T	~~E~~	E	T	C	I	R	M	A	S	I	E	~~N~~	L	O	~~F~~	A	~~W~~	H	A	T	N	T	S	P	R	E	V	N	S
~~B~~	~~A~~	~~C~~	N	E	T	I	A	L	T	~~C~~	O	L	~~Y~~	~~D~~	E	X	I	S	T	B	U	O		P	O	R	I	E	N	T
D	O	~~N~~	~~I~~	~~F~~	R	L	~~D~~	E	N	T	~~R~~	O	N		~~W~~	~~C~~	L	~~L~~	H	I	L	~~G~~
~~P~~	~~H~~		~~C~~	~~C~~		L	I		S		A				~~E~~	~~P~~		~~A~~

ANSWER: _____

Erythromycin, Clindamycin, and Miscellaneous Penicillin Substitutes

Listed below are several of the penicillin substitutes and their characteristics. Some of these characteristics are shared by one or more of the drugs, others are true for only one compound. Match the characteristic with each drug. Use each drug as many times as needed. Some characteristics will have multiple entries.

A. Erythromycin   D. Vancomycin

B. Clindamycin   E. Bacitracin

C. Lincomycin   F. Spectinomycin

_____1. May be given by oral, IM, or IV routes.

_____2. Does not appear in the cerebrospinal fluid of normal patients but may enter the CNS when the meninges are inflamed by infection.

_____3. Extensively biodegraded in the liver; the liver is the primary site of biotransformation. Since less than 20% of the drug shows up as active antibiotic in urine or feces, these drugs are used at normal dosages in patients with renal insufficiency or failure.

_____4. The kidney is the major excretory route.

_____5. May cause deafness in some patients.

_____6. Has a similar antimicrobial spectrum to penicillin G but is chemically unrelated to penicillins and is not cross-allergenic with them.

_____7. Most commonly used against gram-positive bacteria as a topical ointment.

_____8. Inhibits bacterial protein synthesis; both gram-positive and gram-negative bacteria may be affected, but the ability to inhibit _N. gonorrhoeae_ is the basis for clinical usefulness.

_____9. Chemically unrelated to penicillins with a different mechanism of action; will act against organisms that resist penicillins, including methicillin-resistant staphylococci.

_____10. The danger of severe colitis limits use.

TRUE OR FALSE

_____ 11. The drugs known as the macrolides bind to bacterial ribosomes thus preventing bacterial protein synthesis.

_____ 12. Included in the macrolide class are the drugs erythromycin, azithromycin, clindamycin, and clarithromycin.

_____ 13. One of the ways bacteria become resistant to erythromycin is that gram-positive organisms seem to be relatively impermeable to erythromycin and are therefore intrinsically resistant.

_____ 14. Gram-negative organisms chemically alter their ribosomes so that the ribosomes no longer bind to erythromycin; thus protein synthesis is not inhibited.

_____ 15. Erythromycin is sensitive to acid and therefore may be extensively degraded in the stomach.

_____ 16. Food may interfere with the oral absorption of most erythromycin preparations, erythromycin estolate and erythromycin ethylsuccinate being exceptions.

_____ 17. When given parentally, erythromycin gluceptate should be diluted with sterile water for injection and administered intramuscularly.

_____ 18. Erythromycin readily enters body tissues, and tissue concentrations of drug may persist well beyond the point of detection in serum.

_____ 19. Erythromycin is especially concentrated in the liver and spleen. It enters fluids of the middle ear and pleural fluids but not cerebrospinal fluid, unless the meninges are inflamed.

_____ 20. Although erythromycin crosses the placenta, fetal blood levels are less than 20% of maternal blood levels.

_____ 21. Erythromycin enters breast milk but concentrations are much lower than that of maternal serum.

_____ 22. Other macrolides are more strongly concentrated in tissues than erythromycin and therefore persist longer in the body.

_____ 23. The liver is the major excretory organ for erythromycin and other macrolides.

_____ 24. Erythromycin is a useful substitute in patients allergic to penicillin because it has a similar antimicrobial spectrum to penicillin G but is chemically unrelated.

_____ 25. Erythromycin is the drug of choice for atypical pneumonias such as those caused by Mycoplasma pneumonia and Legionella pneumophilia (Legionnaires' disease) .

CHAPTER 32

Tetracyclines and Chloramphenicol

BUBBLES

The answer to each of the clues in this puzzle is a five-letter word related to tetracycline and chloramphenicol. Enter each word into the grid by placing its first letter in the center of the correspondingly numbered bubble, and the remaining letters in the four outer spaces, proceeding clockwise. It's up to you to determine where the outer four letters begin in each bubble. Good luck!

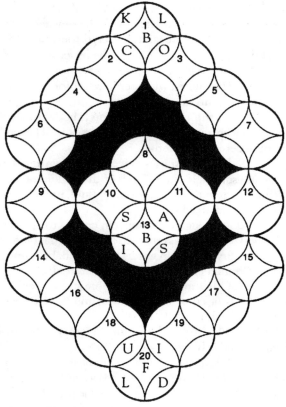

1. The tetracyclines _____ bacterial growth by preventing ribosomes from binding messenger RNA, thereby preventing the initiation of protein synthesis.
2. Tetr_____ines are clinically important because of their wide antibacterial spectrum.
3. Resistant bacterium _____ the ability to transport tetracyclines into the bacterial cell, and the antibiotic does not come in contact with its intracellular target.
4. Absorption of tetracyclines is influenced by an _____ lability, water solubility, and lipid solubility.
5. _____ of chloramphenicol are inactivated in the liver.

6. Chloramphenicol may induce an irreversible bone marrow depression, which _____ to aplastic anemia, a condition with high mortality.
7. Tetracycline _____ effectively when transported into bacterial cells.
8. _____ in the tetracycline family are bacteriostatic rather than bactericidal.
9. Chloramphenicol is the drug of choice for typhoid _____, life-threatening bacteremias, or meningitis.
10. Outdated tetracycline preparations have been implicated in occasional adverse reactions including symptoms of systemic _____ erythematosus.
11. Chloramphenicol inhibits bacterial protein synthesis. The mechanism of action differs from tetracyclines in that chloramphenicol inhibits late rather than _____ steps in ribosomal function.
12. The peak _____ concentration of chloramphenicol achieved by an oral dose is about the same as that produced by an equivalent dose given IV.
13. Families of patients treated on a long-term _____ with low doses of tetracyclines may show a conversion of the normal tetracycline-sensitive bacterial flora to tetracycline-resistant forms.
14. Absorption of tetracyclines from intramuscular _____ is generally poor and frequently causes local tissue irritation and pain at the injection site, therefore limiting its use.
15. Chloramphenicol can inhibit drug-metabolizing enzymes of the liver leading to dangerous interaction with drugs that have a relatively low therapeutic index and _____ route of elimination by microsomal enzymes of the liver.
16. Tetracyclines _____ a wide variety of adverse reactions, most commonly G.I. irritation.
17. Tetracyclines are administered primarily by the oral _____ as a hydrochloride or phosphate salt to increase solubility and thereby increase absorption.
18. Chloramphenicol easily crosses the placenta and appears in _____ milk.
19. Tetracyclines bind to calcium which leads to their deposition in bones and teeth. In adults, this binding produces little visible effect, but in children under eight this will _____ the newly formed permanent teeth.
20. Unlike many other antibiotics, chloramphenicol will enter the cerebrospinal _____ relatively easily, even when the meninges are not inflamed.

Aminoglycosides and Polymyxins

Hidden in each box on this page are five words related to aminoglycosides and polymyxins. Each word or phrase is divided into parts and concealed sequentially from left to right in consecutive columns. Identify, on the blanks below, each word hidden in the accompanying box. Cross out squares as you find each word, because each will be used only once.

A	A	N	G	L
E	E	R	D	T
R	R	N	N	S
B	I	U	L	Y
D	G	E	A	S

1. _____   4. _____

2. _____   5. _____

3. _____

1. Assess _____ function, hearing acuity, and vestibular function before administering aminoglycosides or polymyxins.
2. It is important to note whether the patient to receive an aminoglycoside or polymyxin has been given a neuromuscular _____ or has a condition such as myasthenia gravis that would predispose the patient to respiratory paralysis.
3. The aminoglycosides inhibit _____ steps in bacterial protein synthesis by binding to bacterial ribosomes.
4. Resistance to aminoglycosides may occur because of a decreased antibiotic uptake, a change in the way the antibiotic _____ to the ribosome, or enzymatic destruction of the aminoglycoside.
5. As a result of being charged, the _____ in the aminoglycoside group do not penetrate mammalian membranes readily and are not absorbed orally.

S	I	S	R	E	R
D	Y	G	G	E	M
K	O	T	I	E	E
L	C	D	T	E	Y
A	E	N	N	O	N

6. _____   9. _____

7. _____   10 _____

8. _____

6. Aminoglycosides do not enter the central nervous _____ to any significant extent.
7. Aminoglycosides are excreted by glomerular filtration in the _____.
8. The half-life of the aminoglycosides is much _____ in patients with renal failure than in healthy patients.
9. A difference amony aminoglycosides is their different _____ of activity against *P. aeruginosa*.
10. Polymyxins are of clinical interest because of their bactericidal _____ on gram-negative bacteria.

I	E	A	S
G	R	A	W
C	E	N	K
P	O	L	M
S	L	O	L

11. _____   14. _____

12. _____   15. _____

13. _____

11. Generally, the aminoglycosides are reserved for serious infection caused by aerobic _____-negative bacteria or by mycobacteria.
12. Polymyxins alter the permeability of bacterial cell membranes, causing the loss of required small molecules and _____ from the cell.
13. Organisms naturally resistant to polymyxins possess barriers that prevent polymyxin from contacting the _____ membrane.
14. _____ blood levels are reached about 2 hours after IM injection of polymyxins, but severe pain may result with this route of administration.
15. IV administration of the polymyxins is by relatively _____ infusion.

Sulfonamides, Trimethoprim, Quinolones, and Furantoins

HIDDEN AGENDA

Terms relating to the sulfonamides, trimethoprim, quinolones, and furantoins are hidden in the grid below.
They may appear vertically, horizontally, diagonally, left-
to-right, or right-to-left. First solve the clues below, then
locate each in the grid by either highlighting or circling
the word.

D	Y	S	C	R	A	S	I	A	S	S	T	L	E	T
M	Q	U	I	N	E	C	N	A	T	S	I	S	E	R
A	U	R	I	N	A	R	Y	H	C	G	A	Y	L	I
I	I	A	E	I	C	H	A	M	R	R	D	N	I	M
T	N	K	G	R	R	I	N	A	Y	A	N	E	C	E
I	O	C	A	E	C	N	L	G	M	Y	A	R	R	T
M	L	M	L	L	I	A	C	E	N	H	Y	G	E	H
K	O	A	I	E	N	J	Y	U	K	S	R	I	H	O
I	N	J	T	E	O	A	L	E	T	U	N	S	A	P
D	E	R	R	O	X	P	T	A	H	I	B	T	G	R
N	S	E	A	E	A	I	L	O	A	E	H	I	M	I
E	N	O	C	L	C	S	Z	M	B	A	T	C	T	M
Y	I	E	A	I	I	N	R	S	A	M	S	A	L	P
S	U	L	F	O	N	A	M	I	D	E	S	N	E	S
N	I	T	R	O	F	U	R	A	N	T	O	I	N	P

1. _____ are metabolic inhibitors
that block bacterial synthesis of folic acid.

2. _____ inhibits dihydrofolic acid
reductase and thereby also prevents tetrahydrofolic acid
formation in bacteria.

3. Bacterial _____ to sulfonamides
has become widespread and has reduced their clinical usefulness.

4. Elimination of sulfonamides from the body involves the
liver and the _____.

5. Trimethoprim is combined with sulfamethoxazole in a
1:5 trimethoprim/sulfamethoxazole ratio. This combination is _____.

6. Trimethoprim appears in the urine at a concentration
100 times the _____ concentration with most of
the drug in active form.

7. Deaths from aplastic anemia and other blood
_____, although rare, have been
connected with sulfonamide therapy.

8. _____ interfere
with DNA replication in bacteria by inhibiting the proper
functioning of DNA gyrase.

9. DNA _____ is the enzyme that allows
bacterial DNA to unwind so that replication may proceed.

10. The quinolones include ciprofloxacin, norfloxacin,
_____, nalidixic acid, and enoxacin.

11. Adjust doses of quinolones in patients with
_____ impairment because the kidneys are the primary organ of excretion of active drugs or metabolites.

12. Quinolones are contraindicated in children because
they can permanently damage _____.

13. _____ inhibits cer-
tain bacterial enzymes required for metabolism of sugar
and perhaps other compounds.

14. Although nitrofurantoin is not effective systemically,
it is effective against _____ tract infec-
tions.

15. The gastric irritation associated with nitrofurantoin
administration is reduced if the drug is administered as
large _____ rather than in the original
microcrystalline form.

CHAPTER 35

Drugs to Treat Tuberculosis and Leprosy

TOSSED-WORD PUZZLE

Unscramble the terms below and write them in the blanks to the right to reveal a profile of tuberculosis. Then unscramble the boxed letters to fill in the blank under the clue.

1. f i s u c e n i t o

— — — — — ☐ — — ☐ ☐

2. c a b a r o m y c e i t

— — — — ☐ — — — ☐ ☐ ☐ ☐ —

3. z o c y t a g h i p e

— — — — ☐ ☐ — — — — — —

4. u n e o f l s

☐ ☐ ☐ — — — — —

CLUE: It will take more than the mounties to reign it in because the "white plague" has become

— — — — — — — — — — — — — —

MULTIPLE CHOICE

____ 5. The traditional method of chemotherapy for established tuberculosis has been to administer a combination of drugs for
A. 2 years or longer
B. 2 to 3 months
C. 6 months to 1 year
D. several weeks, until patients cease to be infectious.

____ 6. Tuberculosis and leprosy are diseases produced by
A. norcardia
B. actinomycen
C. mycobacterium
D. chlamydia infections

____ 7. Tuberculosis, or the white plague, was a major cause of death in Europe and the Orient until the _____ when the first antituberculosis agent was introduced.
A. 1900s
B. 1920s
C. 1940s
D. 1960s

____ 8. Antituberculosis therapy is used in patients

A. diagnosed with active TB
B. whose TB skin tests convert from negative to positive
C. receiving high doses of adrenocortical steroids
D. all of the above.

____ 9. ____, the best antituberculosis drug available, is the only agent used alone routinely for prophylaxis.
A. rifampin
B. isoniazid
C. streptomycin
D. ethambutol

____10. When used to treat tuberculosis _____ has the broadest spectrum of activity of all antituberculosis agents, but it is expensive and can cause increased toxicity when administered intermittently.
A. rifampin
B. ethambutol
C. isoniazid
D. sulfone dapsone

____11. _____ is an antituberculosis drug chemically unrelated to other antituberculosis drugs or antibiotics.
A. rifampin
B. isoniazid
C. streptomycin
D. ethambutol

____ 12. _____ was the first antituberculosis drug to be discovered.
A. rifampin
B. isoniazid
C. streptomycin
D. ethambutol

____13. In the past this drug was included in the standard three-drug regimen for TB but it's not well tolerated in most patients and current treatment protocols are more likely to include ethambutol or rifampin.
A. amikacin
B. aminosalicylate
C. ethionamide
D. pyrazinamide

____14. A reserve drug used in the treatment of TB, generally more toxic than first line drugs.
A. amikacin
B. capreomycin
C. cycloserin
D. all of the above

CHAPTER 36

Antifungal Agents

In the puzzles below, you are to fit the letters in each column into the boxes directly above them in order to form words. The letters may or may not go into the boxes in the same order in which they are given. It is up to you to decide which letter goes into which box above it. Once a letter is used, it cannot be used again. A ◆ indicates the end of a word. When the diagram has been filled in, it will be your clue for solving the puzzle.

1.

h	u			n	◆		e	l		◆		c					i		◆
	h	o		e	s			r	o		◆		n	◆				i	
		m	b		a	n		◆		b		◆			u	n		◆
			t				◆	◆	◆	◆	◆	◆	◆	◆	◆	◆	◆	◆
c	h	n	a	r	i	t	e	s	o	b	u	t	n	f	u	n	g	i	r
c	e	m	l	a	a	n	e	r	l	l		i	o	n	t	h	i	i
h	o	m	t	e	s	n	e	l		s		e			t	a	e	n
m	u	o	b	n		c

ANSWER _____

2.

f	u			i	◆	w			s		◆	g		o			h	◆	◆
		◆		a		m		s	t	◆	a	l		a		◆	◆	◆	◆
	s	t		i		t	e		◆		o	◆	h		m		◆
s	k		◆		r		◆	c		l		◆	◆	◆	◆	◆
f	s	s	t	r	m	c	h	t	d	a	l	g	e	h	s	t	h	n
i	u	i	a	t	i	r	e	o	s	e	t	l	a	o	u	m	a
r	k	n	n	l	a	o	s	e	e	a	l	o	r	d	w
s	e		g			w	t				w		y

ANSWER _____

3.

f	u	n				◆			n	f		c					◆
			t	r		c	t		◆		t		◆	s	k		n
◆	m	u			◆	m		m		r		n			,
		◆	g		◆				◆			e	◆	◆	◆
f	r	s	t	a	l	e	r	m	f	m	e	r	a	s	k	s	n
o	u	u	c	r	i	s	i	e	e	e	t	o	i	o	e	i
r	m	n	g	i	u	t	a	c	t	b	t	r	n	s
	e		g	o		n	d			a		e

ANSWER _____

Treatment of Viral Diseases

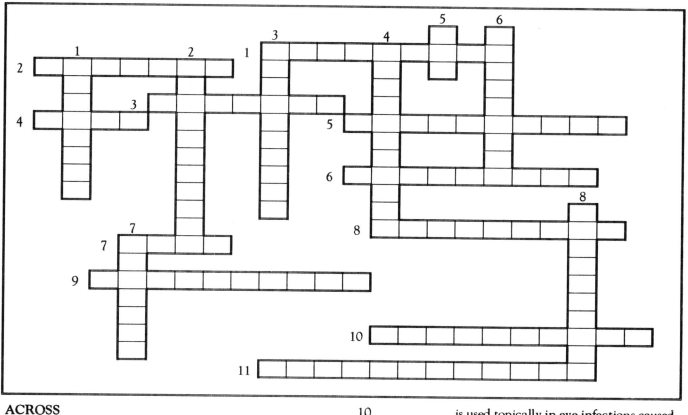

ACROSS

1. The external surface of viruses contains _____ substances that promote antibody production.

2. Some viruses have the potential for more generalized invasion of tissues throughout the body by a mechanism called _____ spread.

3. The most successful immunization programs are for viral diseases in which few pathogenic _____ exist and with which antigenic properties do not change.

4. The activated form of acyclovir preferentially and irreversibly inhibits the viral DNA polymerase present in an infected _____, effectively halting virus production.

5. _____ is a purine analogue that is activated by phosphorylation within cells and in this active form blocks synthesis of HIV DNA.

6. _____ has shown activity against HIV, herpes viruses, and hepatitis B but is presently indicated only for control of CMV retinitis in HIV-infected patients.

7. Interferons are _____ specific, not virus specific.

8. In the U.S., _____ is indicated only for therapy of severe respiratory syncytial virus (RSV) in children.

9. _____ appears to block uncoating of influenza type A viruses and has a narrow antiviral spectrum.

10. _____ is used topically in eye infections caused by herpes but is teratogenic and potentially carcinogenic.

11. _____ is effective for topical therapy of herpes infections of the eye.

DOWN

1. _____ cells are also changed sufficiently in many viral diseases so that these cells are also eliminated.

2. The body limits the spread of viral diseases by the production of glycoproteins called _____.

3. Many viral diseases are best controlled by inducing _____ in healthy individuals before exposure to the viral disease.

4. _____ , like acyclovir, is readily activated within virus-infected cells to a form that inhibits virus reproduction.

5. Retroviruses use _____ as their genetic material.

6. _____, one of the most highly selective of the antiviral agents used in the U.S., is activated by viral thymidine kinase, an enzyme found in only virus-infected cells.

7. _____ factors limit the spread of many types of viral disease and allow the body to eliminate the virus.

8. _____ is used to treat AIDS and AIDS-related complex.

CHAPTER 38

Drugs to Treat Protozoal and Helminthic Infestations

FILL IN THE BLANKS

1. _____ is caused by a microscopic, single-celled parasitic organism.

2. _____ is a frequent pathogen in humans, commonly passed from host to host by oral ingestion of fecally contaminated food or water.

3. In an amebic disease, once in the intestine, the nonmotile cysts change to a motile, sexually active form called a _____.

4. Cryptosporidia are small _____ that can cause diarrhea in several species of animals and humans.

5. Giardiasis is an intestinal infection caused by the protozoan _____.

6. _____ is a serious infectious illness caused when an infected mosquito injects a species of *Plasmodium* into the bloodstream of a person.

7. Although more related to fungi, _____ _____ is more effectively treated with antiprotozoal agents. It can produce severe pulmonary disease in patients receiving immunosuppressive drugs or suffering from AIDS.

8. The most common source of infection with _____ _____ is cat feces.

9. Flukes, tapeworms and roundworms are disease-causing _____.

10. _____ is pinworm infestation.

11. _____ infestation, also called strong lyloidiasis, is more serious than many other infestations because the worm may reproduce in the human body.

12. _____, also known as pork roundworm infestation, is much less common today than it once was.

MATCHING

_____ 13. Member of drug family called 4-aminoquinolines. Mainstay of antimalarial therapy.

_____ 14. Related to emetine, an alkaloid obtained from ipecac. May block protein synthesis in eukaryotes.

_____ 15. Effective amebicidal agent whose action is thought to relate to the iodine content of drug.

_____ 16. Effective broad-spectrum antihelminthic agent, blocks glucose uptake in sensitive helminths.

_____ 17. Chemically related to quinine and acts only against the blood-borne forms of *Plasmodium*.

_____ 18. Attacks amebas at intestinal and other tissue sites, also effective in treating trichomoniasis.

_____ 19. Action of this drug against *P. carinii* is not completely understood but involves an interference with DNA function.

_____ 20. General antiseptic agent; effect is produced by the release of free iodine

_____ 21. Interferes with the function of suckers on cestodes and flukes, thereby causing these parasites to dislodge from tissue sites in the host

_____ 22. Depolarizing neuromuscular blocking agent, similar action to succinylcholine and decamethonium; causes spastic paralysis and gradual contraction of worm muscles.

_____ 23. Inhibits the enzyme dihydrofolate reductase in plasmodia. Blocks formation of THFA.

_____ 24. First developed and used as antimalarial but now primarily used for giardiasis.

_____ 25. Macrolide antibiotic related to erythromycin, most likely affects bacterial ribosomes in the same way as erythromycin.

A. Dehydroemetine

B. Mefloquine

C. Pentamidine

D. Povidone-iodine

E. Pyrantel pamoate

F. Pyrimethamine

G. Metronidazole

H. Iodoquinol

I. Chloroquine

J. Mebendazole

K. Praziquantel

L. Quinacrine

M. Spiramycin

CHAPTER 39

Drugs to Treat Neoplastic Diseases

Hidden in each box on this page are five words related to the treatment of neoplastic diseases. Each word or phrase is divided into five parts and concealed sequentially from left to right in consecutive columns. Identify, on the blanks below, each word hidden in the accompanying box. Cross out squares as you find each word, because each will be used only once.

L	E	N	T
C	O	S	S
M	E	S	L
G	O	L	E
H	A	S	E

1. _____   4. _____

2. _____   5. _____

3. _____

1. Carcinogenesis is the process by which a normal _____ is transformed into a cancerous cell.
2. An oncogene is an altered regulatory _____ associated with cancer.
3. Cancer cells _____ the normal property called contact inhibition.
4. Cancer cells can metastasize, a process in which cancer cells separate from the original _____ and move directly or are carried by blood or lymph to distant sites.
5. In theory, one cancer cell left living in the _____ after therapy is sufficient cause for recurrence.

C	G	T	T	T	G
A	A	S	A	N	S
A	R	N	N	K	S
B	Y	E	C	E	R
S	C	E	I	E	M

6. _____   9. _____

7. _____   10. _____

8. _____

6. A difficulty in treating neoplastic diseases is that _____ cells offer fewer targets for selective toxicity than bacterial cells.
7. Alkylating _____ form highly reactive compounds in the body that react with many chemicals including nucleic acids.

8. Bleomycin is a mixture of glycopeptides derived from cultures of streptomyces. The drug is therefore an antibiotic that produces _____ in DNA strands.
9. Carmustine is a rapidly-acting alkylating agent, and penetrates blood-brain barrier well. It's therefore useful in controlling symptoms produced by tumors of the central nervous _____.
10. Chlorambucil is distinguished by being the slowest _____ and the least toxic of the nitrogen mustard alkylating agents.

A	Y	V	A	T
C	I	C	E	R
L	R	E	L	E
P	G	E	N	T
T	H	A	S	E

11. _____   14. _____

12. _____   15. _____

13. _____

11. Cisplatin and carboplatin cross-link DNA and are not specific for cell _____.
12. Cyclophosphamide is a noncytotoxic form of nitrogen mustard that must be activated by _____ microsomal enzymes.
13. Dacarbazine is used to _____ malignant melanoma and Hodgkin's disease.
14. Mechlorethamine is a potent alkylating _____.
15. Mitoxantrone, used in acute nonlymphocytic leukemia, reacts with DNA by an unknown mechanism; it is not specific for a particular _____ of the cell cycle.

CHAPTER 40

Sedative-Hypnotic Agents, Antianxiety Agents, and Alcohol

BUBBLES

The answer to each of the clues in this puzzle is a five-letter word related to sedative-hypnotic agents, antianxiety agents, and alcohol. Enter each word into the grid by placing its first letter in the center of the correspondingly numbered bubble, and the remaining letters in the four outer spaces, proceeding clockwise. It's up to you to determine where the outer four letters begin in each bubble. Good luck!

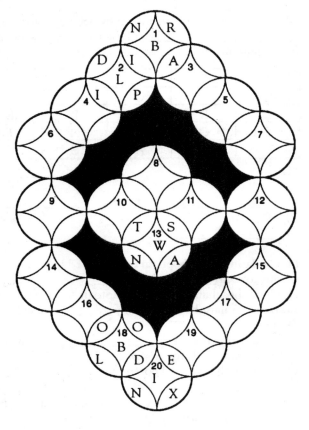

1. Sedative-hypnotic drugs, antianxiety drugs, and alcohol are CNS depressants since they depress the reticular activating system of the _____ stem.
2. Benzodiazepines are highly _____ - soluble and therefore widely distributed in body tissues.
3. At first _____ of CNS depression, sedation is produced, characterized by decreased physical and mental responses to stimuli.
4. More than 50 derivatives of barbituric acid have been marketed for clinical use _____ the beginning of this century, and nine are still widely used.

5. With an increased dose of a CNS depressant, disinhibition is the next _____ of depression reached.
6. The reticular activating system refers to neural pathways in which incoming signals form the senses (sight, sound, smell, _____, taste, and balance) and viscera are collected, processed, and passed on to the higher brain centers.
7. Continued administration of a general-CNS depressant drug can _____ dependence.
8. Buspirone (BuSpar) is a _____ antianxiety drug that is not a benzodiazepine.
9. Benzodiazepines increase the action of the inhibitory neurotransmitter, _____ aminobutyric acid (GABA).
10. _____ alcohol syndrome is characterized by a flat face with widely spaced, small eyes and mental retardation.
11. _____ most popular as a sedative or an antianxiety agent are those that produce minimal sleepiness at an effective dose.
12. An increased incidence of _____ lip has been reported among infants whose mothers took diazepam (Valium) during early pregnancy.
13. Disulfiram, which blocks the oxidation of acetaldehyde, is prescribed for the detoxified patient who _____ to avoid drinking again.
14. Physical dependence can be overcome by decreasing the drug intake by 10% of the initial dose _____ for 10 days.
15. A butabarbital-_____ is frequently used to treat conditions with psychogenic overtones such as allergies, ulcers, and inflammatory bowel disease.
16. Benzodiazepines are contraindicated for women in _____ and for nursing mothers because of adverse depression of the infant.
17. The most common pattern of cross-tolerance, a major factor in drug _____, is alcohol in combination with one or more sedative-hypnotic or anti-anxiety drugs.
18. Barbiturates are released slowly from muscle and fat into the _____ for eventual metabolism by the liver and excretion by the kidney.
19. Although chloral hydrate (Noctec) is not effective for more than 2 _____, it does not suppress REM sleep and therefore doesn't cause REM rebound.
20. Benzodiazepines rapidly gained popularity and acceptance because of their high therapeutic _____.

40

CHAPTER 41

Antipsychotic Drugs

COMPLETE THE STATEMENT

1. _____ refers to the ability of antipsychotic drugs to cause a general quiescence and a state of psychic indifference to the surroundings.

2. Three major uses of antipsychotic drugs are

_____

_____

_____

3. _____ is a major emotional disorder with an impairment of mental function great enough to prevent the individual from participating in everyday life.

4. _____ may be an isolated "breakdown" caused by a major traumatic event.

5. _____ is a chronic mental illness with psychotic episodes.

6. An _____ results from damage to the brain by infectious diseases, deficiency diseases, lead poisoning, tumors, and injury through trauma or interrupted blood supply such as in cerebrovascular accidents.

7. _____ can arise during withdrawal from alcohol or other drugs.

8. The five chemical classes of antipsychotic drugs are

_____

_____

_____

_____

_____

9. The phenothiazines are subdivided into three subgroups based on chemical differences in side groups on the three-ringed main structure. The subgroups are

_____

_____

_____

10. The four effects of antipsychotic drugs which have been linked to the blockade of dopamine receptors in various parts of the brain are

_____

_____

_____

_____

11. One of the common extrapyramidal effects caused by antipsycotic drugs is

_____

12. _____ is the neurotransmitter in the medullary chemoreceptor trigger zone involved in vomiting.

13. Antipsychotic effects may not be seen for _____ after the start of therapy and _____ are needed to see the full effect of a given dosage regimen.

14. _____ is a spasm of muscles of the tongue, face, neck, or back and may mimic seizures.

15. _____ is a motor restlessness and may be mistaken for psychotic restlessness or agitation.

16. _____ is marked by motor retardation and rigidity.

17. _____, the worst of the extrapyramidal reactions, is associated with long-term, high-dose antipsychotic therapy.

18. Endocrine disturbances in women that are associated with antipsychotic drugs include delayed ovulation and menstruation, amenorrhea, _____ or weight gain.

19. A _____ , the depression of the synthesis of one of the blood elements, occasionally occurs with antipsychotic therapy.

20. Antipsychotic drugs _____ the action of CNS depressant drugs, including sedative-hypnotic drugs, narcotic analgesics, and anesthetic agents.

CHAPTER 42

Antidepressant Drugs

TOSSED-WORD PUZZLE
Unscramble the words below. Then unscramble the boxed letters to fill in the blank under the clue.

1. n e c r o x t i e

   __ ☐ __ __ __ __ ☐ __ ☐ __

2. c n a i m

   __ __ __ ☐ ☐ __

3. c i c c i r t l y

   __ __ __ __ ☐ __ __ ☐ __ __

4. i n t o r a c e

   __ __ __ __ ☐ __ __ __

CLUE: The therapeutic index of lithium is small; monitor plasma levels frequently to avoid

__ __ __ __ __ __ __

MULTIPLE CHOICE

5. _____ is a disorder of mood that occurs in an estimated 15% to 30% of all adults at some time during their lives.

A. depression   C. endogenous depression
B. reaction depression   D. manic depressive disorder

6. _____ is experienced after some significant loss in life.

A. depression   C. endogenous depression
B. reaction depression   D. manic depression

7. A depression with no apparant cause is called _____.

A. depression   C. endogenous depression
B. reaction depression   D. manic depressive disorder

8. _____ is characterized by a manic period with excessive euphoria, self confidence, and little need for sleep, alternating with a period of depression.

A. depression   C. endogenous depression
B. reaction depression   D. manic depressive disorder

9. _____ blocks the reuptake of norepinephrine or serotonin into the presynaptic neurons.

A. MAO inhibitor   C. lithium
B. tricyclic antidepressant   D. antipsychotic drug

10. Tricyclic antidepressants exert _____ action on the heart.
A. anticholinergic   C. quinidine-like action
B. adrenolytic   D. all of the above

MATCHING

11. _____ block the reuptake of norepinephrine or serotonin into presynaptic neurons.
12. _____(Elavil), a tricyclic antidepressant, is associated with a high incidence of sedation and anticholinergic effects.
13. _____ (Adapin and Sinequan) does not have the quinidine-like cardiac effect that other tricyclic antidepressants have; indicated when cardiac function must be considered.
14. _____(Vivactil) is a tricyclic antidepressant with minimum sedating effect.
15. Drugs that are neither tricyclics nor MAO inhibitors, _____ have a lesser incidence of anticholinergic side effects, less cardiotoxicity, and faster onset of action than tricyclics.
16. _____ (Ascendin) inhibits amine uptake and is a more potent inhibitor of norepinephrine than serotonin.
17. _____ (Prozac) is a newer antidepressant, less likely to cause anticholinergic effects.
18. _____ are effective because they prevent degradation of norepinephrine and serotonin so that concentration of CNS neurotransmitters is increased.
19. _____(Nardil) is the safest MAO inhibitor.
20. _____ is the drug of choice for treating the manic phase of manic-depressive disorder.

A. phenelzine
B. second-generation antidepressants
C. doxepin
D. tricyclic antidepressants
E. amoxapine
F. fluoxetine
G. lithium
H. MAO inhibitors
I. amitriptyline
J. protriptyline

Central Nervous System Stimulants

In the puzzles below, you are to fit the letters in each column into the boxes directly above them in order to form words. The letters may or may not go into the boxes in the same order in which they are given. It is up to you to decide which letter goes into which box above it. Once a letter is used, it cannot be used again. A ♦ indicates the end of a word. When the diagram has been filled in, it will be your clue for solving the puzzle.

1.

P	C	T	D	D	L	T	A	U	N	E	A	P	E	C	T	E	D	H	Y
A	A	I	I	E	I	Y	S	F	E	X	P	N	I	R	M	A	L	E	
	M	A	L	L	N	T		O	L		E			O	N		T	L	
	F	T	I	V	S														

ANSWER: _____

2.

S	H	S	P	F	T	S	M	U	M	O	P	T	S	I	T	H	A	T
W	U	I	L	E	E	N	S	I	A	P	L	E	T	I	N	E		
C	N	P	R	U	I	T	T	I	U	N	A	T	T	G				
C	N	S	S	S	C	L	A	N	S									

ANSWER_____

3.

S	E	S	P	S	L	A	T	E	T	T	I	S	S	L	T	O	T	I	O	N
P	X	U	E	O	N	S	H	V	S	R	I	M	C	I	I	A	S	N	D	
R	T	I	M	U	N	A	I	A	E	N	E	N	U	R	R	A	A	E		
E	R	T	G	R		T	L			E	S	P		E						

ANSWER_____

Narcotic Analgesics (Opioids)

```
F R U O P I O I D S U M T Y D B
E B R B N E E A N D O E R I Y U
S U B J E C T I V E C T I K N T
T A N E S T H E S I A H G S O O
N A R C A N T A N Y G A G N R R
Y R O T A R I P S E R D E I P P
A D D I C T I O N I C O R L H H
T C N V B T E S L I V N Z A I A
W I D E Z O C I N E O E O H N N
I N I H P R O D N E H W N P S O
A O D A R V O N Z G V I E E L L
N R E T R O H S U P R A L K I G
Y H O U V R C O D E I N E N E L
A C U T E R C S T T J Y A E U K
B U P R E N O R P H I N E H E I
```

1. Morphine is the prototype for the narcotic analgesics, a class of drugs called the _____.

2. Pain is classified into two major conponents: _____ and _____ pain.

3. In treating _____ pain, opioids are administered in sufficient doses to relieve pain and at intervals frequent enough to prevent the recurrence of pain.

4. There is little danger of producing _____ when treating acute pain because psychologic dependence in opioids is unlikely to occur.

5. Opioids treat the _____ pain associated with cancer.

6. The combination of opioid, nitrous oxide, and muscle relaxant is called balanced _____.

7. Beta _____ is a large peptide derived from the prohormone for adrenocorticotropic hormone and is found in the pituitary gland.

8. The _____ are also peptides derived from a larger peptide and found in the pituitary.

9. The _____ are pentapeptides and seem to be neurotransmitters associated with mediation of pain and analgesia; release of

growth hormone prolactin and vasopressin from the pituitary; modulation of locomotor activity; regulation of mood; regulation of gut motility.

Morphine affects these medullary centers:

10. _____

11. _____

12. _____

13. _____ (Dalgan), a new chemically different opiod that relieves pain as effectively as morphine, will not adversely affect cardiac performance.

14. _____ substitutes for other opiods in drug-dependent individuals and prevents withdrawal symptoms.

15. _____ (Buprenex), an opioid with agonist and antagonist properties administered intramuscularly, has a low potential for abuse.

16. The actions of _____ (Stadol) resemble those of morphine, except this drug increases pulmonary arterial pressure and the cardiac workload, making it undesirable for treating the pain of a myocardial infarction.

17. Meperidine (Demerol), the first synthetic narcotic analgesic, has a _____ duration of action than morphine and does not have an antitussive effect.

18. _____ is not administered in doses large enough to be effective as morphine, since the high dose required to produce an equal degree of analgesia results in a high incidence of side effects.

19. Propoxyphene (_____), an opioid related to methadone, is not a very potent analgesic.

20. Naloxone (_____) is a pure antagonist for the opioid receptor, making it especially useful in the emergency room.

CHAPTER 45

General Anesthetics

MATCHING

_____ 1. Gases or volatile liquids administered as gases. Effective concentration does not depend on solubility of the anesthetic in blood or tissue.

_____ 2. Has a wide margin of safety and few cardiovascular effects. But this volatile liquid is flammable, explosive, and unpleasant to inhale because of its noxious pungent order.

_____ 3. A halogenated hydrocarbon and a nonflammable liquid that produces muscle contractions and seizure-like brain waves at high concentrations.

_____ 4. Currently the most widely used volatile liquid anesthetic. A direct myocardial depressant causing a dose-dependant reduction in cardiac output with no change in heart rate.

_____ 5. Nonflammable liquid halogenated hydrocarbon. Produces analgesia adequate for dentistry and obstetrics. Depresses the cardiovascular system but does not sensitize heart to catecholamines.

_____ 6. A nonexplosive gas widely used alone in dental and obstetric procedures and as one component in balanced anesthesia

_____ 7. Drugs used primarily as induction agents to bypass stage II anesthesia.

_____ 8. Produces a cataleptic anesthesia, abolishing perception of and reaction to pain.

_____ 9. Thiopental, methohexital, and thiamylal are ultrashort-acting _____ used to induce anesthesia.

_____ 10. _____ is a benzodiazepine used occasionally as an induction agent but more frequently to sedate patients undergoing cardioversion, endoscopic, or dental procedures.

_____ 11. Relatively short-acting benzodiazepine used as an IV anesthetic. Use only in hospital setting where respiration and cardiac function can be monitored.

_____ 12. _____ is an IV anesthetic for induction of surgical anesthesia. Produces minimum cardiovascular or respiratory changes. Does not produce analgesia.

_____ 13. A new anesthetic for induction and maintenance of general anesthesia. Recovery is rapid with minimal psychomotor impairment.

A. Etomidate	H. Nitrous oxide
B. Diazepam	I. Methoxyflurane
C. Inhalation anesthetics	J. Enflurane
D. Halothane	K. Intravenous Anesthetics
E. Diethyl ether	L. Barbiturates
F. Propofol	M. Ketamine
G. Midazolam	

TRUE OR FALSE

_____ 14. General anesthetics act by a receptor mechanism to abolish the perception of pain and reaction to painful stimuli.

_____ 15. General anesthetics also alter the lipid structure of cell membranes so that physiologic functions are impaired.

_____ 16. The disadvantage of inhalation anesthetics is their slow onset of action.

_____ 17. The potency of an inhalation anesthetic is determined by the minimum alveolar contraction (MAC) that produces insensitivity to a skin incision in 75% of patients.

_____ 18. Distribution of the anesthetic is determined by blood flow, thus the brain, liver, and kidneys reach equilibrium first.

_____ 19. Excretion of inhalation anesthetics is largely through the kidneys.

_____ 20. The time during which the patient regains consciousness after the anesthetic has been discontinued is called emergence.

Local Anesthetics

Hidden in each box on this page are five words related to local anesthetics. Each word or phrase is divided into parts and concealed sequentially from left to right in consecutive columns. Identify, on the blanks below, each word hidden in the accompanying box. Cross out squares as you find each word, because each will be used only once.

B	I	R	A	E
F	L	O	S	T
A	E	R	V	K
N	O	U	S	L
L	B	C	C	E

1. _____   4. _____

2. _____   5. _____

3. _____

1. Local anesthetics reversibly _____ nerve conduction, leading to loss of sensation and preventing muscle activity.
2. In addition to topical anesthesia, local anesthetics can be infiltrated to various _____ sites, producing anesthesia over a wide area.
3. Cocaine was the _____ local anesthetic used clinically, after the observation in the late 1880s that when cocaine was administered orally to patients, their tongues and throats became numb.
4. It was quickly realized that cocaine had a high _____ potential and the drug was replaced by procain (Novocain) by 1905.
5. Lidocaine, introduced in the 1940s, is the most versatile and widely used _____ anesthetic.

R	I	I	E	R
M	A	B	O	D
F	O	P	E	S
P	R	S	I	R
B	A	T	O	R

6. _____   9. _____

7. _____   10. _____

8. _____

6. With administration of local anesthetics, all neurons in the area (whether pain, _____ or autonomic) are affected, so in addition to pain loss, loss of sensory, motor, and autonomic activities occurs.

7. The size of nerve _____ determines its sensitivity to local anesthetics; smaller fibers are the most sensitive.
8. Chemically, most local anesthetics are weak _____, being secondary or tertiary amines.
9. The relative safety of procaine and chloroprocaine results from their _____ hydrolysis in the plasma by pseudocholinesterases.
10. A high plasma concentration of a local anesthetic causes CNS depression, with or without _____ symptoms of CNS stimulation.

S	P	U	D	R	L
S	O	R	U	M	L
V	U	L	A	A	E
S	A	T	U	Y	E
C	P	I	N	A	S

11. _____   14. _____

12. _____   15. _____

13. _____

11. Surface anesthetics are local anesthetics applied as drops, _____, lotions, creams, or ointments.
12. Infiltration anesthesia refers to the superficial application of a local anesthetic. To _____ or cut or to perform dental procedures, local anesthetic is injected in small amounts to block small nerves and numb the area.
13. Nerve block anesthesia refers to the injection of a local anesthetic alone, a nerve before it reaches the surgical site. Both _____ and concentration must be larger than infiltration anesthetic.
14. _____ anesthesia is another form of epidural anesthesia and is achieved by administering the local anesthetic epidurally at the base of the spine.
15. _____ anesthesia is achieved by injecting local anesthetic into subarachnoid space between the arachnoid and pia mater membranes in the lumbar area.

Anticonvulsants

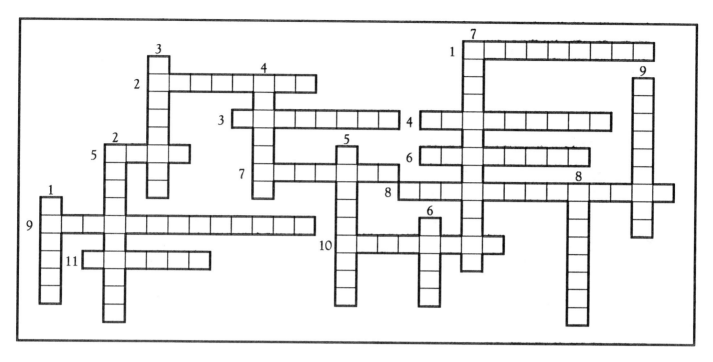

Across

1. _____, formerly called diphenylhydantoin, is a drug of choice in controlling grand mal and focal motor epilepsy in adults.

2. Neurological disorder characterized by recurrent pattern of abnormal neuronal discharges within the brain, resulting in a sudden loss or disturbance of consciousness.

3. Seizure that involves contraction of all skeletal muscles.

4. Generalized seizure pattern considered a genetic disorder (progressive _____ epilepsy).

5. Pre-seizure sensation peculiar to a specific patient.

6. _____ (Valium) is an IV drug of choice for terminating grand-mal seizures of status epilepticus.

7. Petit mal or _____ epilepsy occurs mainly in children, ages 4 to 12.

8. _____ (Tegretol) is particularly effective in controlling seizures of psychomotor and clonic-tonic epilepsy.

9. First drug effective in controlling absence epilepsy, but now a third-choice drug for petit-mal seizures because of serious side effects.

10. _____ lobe or psychomotor epilepsy has complex symptoms including an aura, automatism, and motor seizures, independently or in combination.

11. _____ epilepticus refers to seizures that last 30 min or longer or that are repeated for 30 min or longer and during which consciousness is not regained.

Down

1. Side effects of diazepam include drowsiness, dizziness, and _____.

2. _____ may consist of chewing or swallowing motions, temperament changes, confusion, feelings of unreality, or unexplained, bizarre behavior.

3. Generalized _____ result from discharge of cells over both sides of the brain.

4. _____ seizures arise from a focal lesion of the brain in which the abnormal discharge of cells involves a limited area.

5. _____ spasms denote a major generalized seizure that occurs in the first year of life.

6. _____ seizures are not associated with a loss of consciousness.

7. _____ (Luminal) has been widely used for 60 years and is a drug of choice for grand mal and focal seizures.

8. Nystagmus, an adverse effect of phenytoin, is involuntary movement of the _____.

9. _____ epilepsy is a generalized seizure pattern that develops secondary to anoxic brain damage or as a genetic disorder.

CHAPTER 48

Drugs for Parkinsonism and Centrally Acting Skeletal Muscle Relaxants

MATCHING

_____ 1. A classic anticholinergic drug used to treat Parkinson symptoms for many years.

_____ 2. A synthetic anticholinergic drug that is centrally active and produces fewer peripheral side effects.

_____ 3. Antihistamine used to treat Parkinson's disease.

_____ 4. Antiviral agent effective in reducing severity of Parkinson's symptoms when used alone or in combination with other drugs.

_____ 5. Mimics action of dopamine in the brain.

_____ 6. Inhibits the conversion of levodopa to dopamine.

_____ 7. When other drugs can no longer adequately relieve symptoms of Parkinson's disease, _____ is administered.

_____ 8. Newly approved drug that inhibits the enzyme monoamine oxidase B, which degrades dopamine in the brain.

_____ 9. A benzodiazepine effective in relieving spasticity associated with spinal cord injury, multiple sclerosis, and cerebral injury and in treating muscle spasms.

_____ 10. Analogue of the inhibitory neurotransmitter GABA most effective in relieving spasticity secondary to spinal cord injury.

A. baclofen

B. diphenhydramine

C. bromocriptine

D. carbidopa-levodopa

E. selegiline

F. atropine

G. benztropine

H. levodopa

I. diazepam

J. amantadine

TRUE OR FALSE

_____ 11. Parkinson's disease is a movement disorder characterized by rigidity, akinesia, and tremor.

_____ 12. The current understanding of Parkinson's disease is that it represents a deficiency in the neurotransmitter dopamine in certain basal ganglia.

_____ 13. When dopamine is excessive, muscle tone increases because of the unopposed action of acelylcholine, resulting in muscular rigidity, inhibition of spontaneous movements, and tremor.

_____ 14. Today, the pharmacologic treatment of Parkinson's disease is to diminish the severity of motor symptoms by blocking the excessive action of acetylcholine or by blocking dopamine to return the balance of dopamine and acetylcholine to normal.

_____ 15. Spasticity results from the loss of inhibitory tone in the polysynaptic pathways of the spinal cord so that fine control of motor activity is lost.

CHAPTER 49

Introduction to Endocrinology

BUBBLES

Enter each answer into the grid by placing its first letter in the center of the correspondingly numbered bubble, and the remaining letters in the four outer spaces, proceeding clockwise.

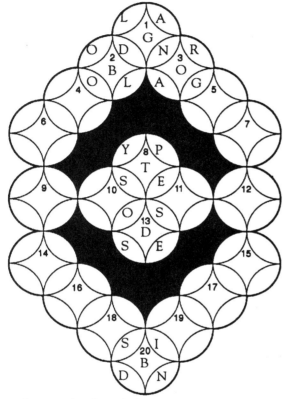

1. The endocrine glands include the pancreas, adrenal glands, thyroid _____, parathyroid glands, testes, ovaries, neurohypophysis, and adenohypophysis.

2. Vasopressin is very rapidly destroyed by enzymes in the _____.

3. Diagnostic hormones assess the function of the target _____ of the administered hormone.

4. The body can _____ several hormones after synthesis for later release.

5. A hormone is a potent _____ capable of exerting profound effects on metabolism.

6. The hormone insulin is degraded in the kidneys and _____.

7. Hormones disappear from the bloodstream when they are taken up by an _____ or when they are degraded by enzymes in the blood.

8. A hormone is a substance produced by cell _____, which act on other cells in the body to produce a physiologic or biochemical response.

9. Replacement therapy is _____ at restoring normal levels of hormones which a patient's body no longer produces.

10. The active _____ of many protein hormones are derived from larger protein molecules called prohormones.

11. The response of target _____ to hormones depends on the number and availability of hormone receptors.

12. The steroid hormones are _____ by soluble receptors, which transport the hormones through the cytoplasm of the cell and into the cell nucleus.

13. How rapidly a hormone is lost from the body determines _____ and dosage schedules.

14. Hormones are used clinically in one of _____ ways: as diagnostic agents, in replacement therapy, or as pharmacologic agents.

15. The second class of hormones is formed from amino _____.

16. Growth hormone is a protein hormone used to _____ a rare endocrine disease.

17. One _____ of hormones is the steroid hormones, which are derived from cholesterol.

18. The time of appearance and the concentration of a hormone in the blood may be regulated by controlling its rate of synthesis, release from storage _____, degradation, and clearance from the body.

19. Hormones may be divided into two classes on the _____ of their chemical composition.

20. Thyroid hormones are transported to the nucleus by nonspecific proteins; in the nucleus the thyroid hormone _____ to specific receptors and ultimately alters protein synthesis in the cell.

Drugs Affecting the Pituitary Gland

TOSSED-WORD PUZZLE

Unscramble the terms below and write them in the blanks to reveal the answers to this clue: In addition to physiologic controls, certain drugs also influence ADH secretion—the following cause release in healthy subjects. Then unscramble the boxed letters to fill in the blank under the second clue.

1. C O T N N E I I

_ _ _ _ _ ☐ _

2. E N I O R P M H

_ ☐ _ _ _ _ _

3. S A T E R U R B A B I T

_ ☐ _ _ _ ☐ _ _ _ _ _

4. C T L H L N E A E Y C O I

_ _ ☐ _ _ _ _ ☐ _ ☐ _ _ _

CLUE: This substance may promote diuresis by inhibiting ADH release

__ __ __ __ __ __ __

COMPLETE THE STATEMENT

5. The posterior pituitary, or _____,
is composed of nerve fibers embryologically derived from the hypothalamus.

6. If the _____ stalk is damaged transportation of the secretory granules to the neurohypophysis is impaired, interfering with release of hormones into the circulation.

7. Antidiuretic hormone is also known as:

_____

8. The primary target tissue of antidiuretic hormone is

_____

9. When ADH is markedly reduced or absent, urine concentration is impossible, and large volumes of dilute, sugar-free urine are produced. This condition is known as

_____

10. Since ADH is a peptide hormone, that cannot be administered orally, and all replacement therapy with ADH involves the administration of the hormone

_____

11. The symptoms of diabetes insipidus may also arise if the neurohypophysis is producing normal amounts of ADH, but the kidney is unresponsive. This syndrome is called _____.

12. Major target organs of _____ are breast myoepithelium and smooth muscles of the uterus, especially during the second and third stages of labor.

13. The anterior pituitary, or _____, constitutes approximately 75% by weight of the pituitary gland and is the master gland of the endocrine system.

14. _____
regulates the length of the long bones in the skeleton, which determines adult stature.

15. Many of the actions of growth hormone are mediated by peptides called _____.

16. Damage to the hypophysis may cause it to produce insufficient quantities of hypophyseal hormones, a condition called _____.

17. Both gigantism and acromegaly usually are caused by pituitary _____, which secrete excessive amounts of growth hormone.

The gonadotropic hormones of the adenohypophysis are

18. _____,

19. _____,

20. _____.

CHAPTER 51

Drugs Affecting the Adrenal Gland

MATCHING

_____ 1. Overproduction of cortisol

_____ 2. Sodium-retaining activity associated with potassium loss

A. Metyrapon

_____ 3. Metabolic effects on carbohydrate, protein, and fat metabolism; antiinflammatory and immunosuppressive activity

B. Cushing's syndrome

C. glucocorticoid action

_____ 4. Synthetic glucocorticoids that are essentially free of mineralocorticoid activity

D. cortisol, cortisone, corticosterone

E. betamethasone, dexamethasone

_____ 5. Natural adrenal steroids

F. mineralocorticoid action

_____ 6. The highly potent synthetic glucocorticoid that is also used diagnostically to test steroid suppression of cortisol synthesis

G. dexamethasone

_____ 7. Blocks cortisol synthesis in adrenal gland and may be used to test the ability of the hypophysis to increase ACTH release

FILL IN THE BLANKS

The two distinct functional units of the human adrenal gland:

8._____

9._____

The two regions of the adrenal gland differ in three distinct ways. Name them:

10._____

11._____

12._____

13. The outer layers or zona glomerulosa of the adrenal cortex is the site of conversion of the precursor cholesterol to the _____.

14. Regulation of mineralocorticoid synthesis is primarily through the _____ .

15. The inner two layers of the _____ convert cholesterol to glucocorticoids and the sex steroids.

16. What are the symptosms of acute adrenal insufficiency?

_____

_____

17. Chronic primary adrenal insufficiency is called

_____ .

CHAPTER 52

Drugs Affecting the Thyroid and Parathyroid Glands

Hidden in each box on this page are five words related to drugs affecting the thyroid and parathyroid glands. Each word or phrase is divided into five parts and concealed sequentially from left to right in consecutive columns. Identify, on the blanks below, answers to the correspondingly numbered question. Then find each word hidden in the accompanying box.

F	L	S	E	L
G	E	T	A	S
A	A	A	H	A
A	F	P	N	R
B	L	T	U	D

1. _____ 4. _____

2. _____ 5. _____

3. _____

1. The thyroid _____ is a richly vascularized, horseshoe-shaped structure lying across the trachea in the larynx region.

2. The function of the follicular cells of the thyroid is to regulate the _____ metabolic rate.

3. Once in the blood most of the thyroid hormones are bound to a special _____ globulin called thyroid-binding globulin.

4. Hypothyroidism may develop in the _____ when a pregnant woman receives antithyroid drugs.

5. Hypothyroidism that develops _____ the neonatal period but before puberty is called juvenile hypthyroidism.

S	O	A	E	R	E
E	R	C	V	E	S
I	E	D	E	G	E
C	H	V	N	N	E
G	X	A	I	S	S

6. _____ 9. _____

7. _____ 10. _____

8. _____

6. The _____ form of hypothyroidism is called myxedema.

7. Hyperthyroidism occurs whenever _____ thyroid hormones are released into the circulation.

8. Hyperthyroidism without thyroid nodules is the most common form of the disease and is referred to as toxic diffuse goiter of _____ disease.

9. Hyperthyroidism most often is controlled with drugs or radioactive _____.

10. Propranolol represents the drug class that controls the symptoms of hyperthyroidism but produces no significant long-term _____ in thyroid hormone levels.

P	C	R	I	I	E
I	O	G	I	A	S
A	A	I	E	N	N
N	R	T	M	O	L
C	O	D	S	T	S

11. _____ 14. _____

12. _____ 15. _____

13. _____

11. Thioamide _____ on the thyroid gland is immediate, and reduced hormone synthesis can be demonstrated within hours.

12. Calcitonin has been used to treat _____ disease, in which excessive bone resorption leads to thinned and fragile bones.

13. The use of radioactive _____ allows the thyroid to be destroyed without resorting to surgery.

14. Iodine may be used as part of emergency therapy for hyperthyroid _____.

15. Treatment of hypothyroidism requires replacement therapy with thyroid hormones to produce the euthyroid state (_____ thyroid hormone levels).

Drugs Acting on the Female Reproductive System

TRUE OR FALSE

_____ 1. The hypothalamus supplies gonadotropin-releasing hormone, a peptide that acts directly on the anteriohypophysis, stimulating synthesis and release of follicle-stimulating hormone and luteinizing hormone.

_____ 2. Under the influence of FSH, ovarian cells synthesize the potent steroid estrogen known as estradiol.

_____ 3. Progestins are compounds that stimulate female reproductive tissues.

_____ 4. Estrogens are compounds that specifically stimulate uterine lining.

_____ 5. Progesterone, the most important progestin, is synthesized in the cells remaining in the follicle after the expulsion of ovum.

_____ 6. At birth the ovary is barely developed; advanced development will not begin until puberty.

_____ 7. A few days after implantation of the ovum in the endometrium, fetal cells begin to produce a hormone called human chorionic gonadotropin.

_____ 8. Prostaglandins, which are hormones formed from fatty acids within cell membranes, are capable of stimulating powerful uterine contractions.

_____ 9. Oxytocin, a hormone produced by the neurohypophysis, is also capaple of inducing contractions.

_____ 10. Many conditions of the female reproductive tract for which women seek medical aid may be treated successfully by replacement therapy. The most common conditons arise from progesterone deficiency.

MATCHING

_____ 11.Induce contraction of the myometrium. Drug class named for the natural neurohypophysis hormone oxytocin.

_____ 12. Class of natural hormones that is involved in regulating myometrial activity.

_____ 13. The best beta-2-adrenergic agonist for use in halting premature labor.

_____ 14. _____, an inhibitor of oxytocin release and a CNS depressant, has been used to halt premature labor.

_____ 15. Preferred general anesthetic to relax uterus, may slow catecholamine release from the adrenal gland.

_____ 16. The natural steroidal compound that normally functions as a uterine relaxant. Use is not recommended in cases of uterine hypertonicity during delivery.

A. ritodrine

B. oxytocic drugs

C. progesterone

D. ethanol

E. halothane

F. prostaglandins

Drugs Acting on the Male Reproductive System

HIDDEN AGENDA

Terms relating to the male reproductive system are hidden in the grid below. They may appear vertically, horizontally, diagonally, left-to-right, or right-to-left. First solve the clues below to fill in the blanks. Then locate each in the grid by either highlighting or circling it.

A	D	R	O	G	E	N	S	T	L	Q	P
N	A	U	R	R	I	Q	N	U	E	I	S
D	N	M	A	O	E	U	O	B	Y	N	T
R	A	D	L	E	J	I	L	U	D	I	T
O	Z	I	L	N	S	E	N	L	I	I	S
G	O	N	Y	E	J	B	O	E	G	A	T
E	L	N	T	L	P	S	B	S	H	A	H
N	T	S	A	E	R	B	A	T	S	P	W
S	E	A	N	A	B	O	L	I	C	P	Y
T	E	S	T	O	S	T	E	R	O	N	E
L	U	T	E	I	N	I	Z	I	N	G	T
C	L	I	M	A	C	T	E	R	I	C	E
K	I	E	N	H	I	S	T	S	H	E	M
O	B	S	T	Y	W	O	N	Y	D	E	R
F	I	U	P	P	L	M	A	N	N	O	N
E	D	P	R	O	L	A	C	T	I	N	A
R	O	T	I	P	H	G	R	H	R	A	N
T	H	I	A	H	M	A	L	E	O	N	G
U	N	D	P	Y	H	A	P	T	V	P	Y
L	I	F	I	S	H	S	C	I	E	I	W
I	T	H	S	I	J	O	Y	C	L	O	L
V	E	M	M	S	E	T	E	L	H	T	A

1. Major reproductive hormones in men.

_____

2. Androgens are synthesized primarily in the _____ and adrenal glands.

3. During fetal development, _____ cells develop in the embryonic testes as a result of stimulation with the maternal hormone, human chorionic gonadotropin.

4. The major steroid affecting male sexual function

_____

5. _____, a weak androgen, is used to suppress LH and FSH release from the hypophysis and to block steroidogenesis.

6. Androgens are still indicated for treatment of certain _____ carcinomas.

7. Unlike testosterone in its natural form methyltestosterone and fluoxymesterone can be administered in this manner: _____

8. Patients who have suffered extensive burns or surgery may benefit from the action of _____ steroids.

9. The seminiferous _____ contain the germ cells that in the adult male produce functional sperm.

10. Interstitial cell-stimulating hormone is also called _____ hormone.

11. Androgen loss after puberty may cause a loss in _____.

12. Male menopause.

13. One type of unresponsiveness to androgens has very high blood levels of _____.

14. Androgens are anabolic (i.e., they stimulate _____ rather than degradative processes.)

15. Bromocriptine increases testosterone and _____ and FSH levels.

16. Continuous penile erection.

17. Prolactin seems to suppress synthesis and release of ICSH and FSH from the _____.

18. Anabolic steroids are inappropriate for use in _____; they run the risk of altered _____ function.

Drugs to Treat Diabetes Mellitus

Hidden in each box on this page are five words related to the treatment of diabetes mellitus. Each word or phrase is divided into five parts and concealed sequentially from left to right in consecutive columns. Identify, on the blanks below, the correct answers to the correspondingly numbered questions. Then find each word hidden in the accompanying box. Cross out squares as you find each word, because each will be used only once.

N	N	V	E	R
C	I	S	E	T
L	E	H	L	R
O	T	L	D	S
O	I	D	E	M

1. _____   4. _____

2. _____   5. _____

3. _____

1. The primary hormone regulating glucose metabolism is insulin, a peptide hormone synthesized in the B _____ of the pancreas.
2. Insulin stimulates glucose uptake in fat and muscle cells and the conversion in the _____ of glucose to storage carbohydrate glycogen.
3. Insulin's metabolic actions must always be considered in relation to the actions of _____ hormones.
4. If all insulin production ceases, the disease is referred to as insulin-dependent diabetes mellitus (IDDM), this form is also called juvenile _____ diabetes
5. If insulin production continues but is insufficient the disease is referred to as noninsulin-dependent diabetes mellitus (_____).

P	B	I	N	O
O	A	E	N	Y
E	C	C	S	R
A	M	R	U	E
O	R	O	L	E

6. _____   9. _____

7. _____   10. _____

8. _____

6. NIDDM is usually a disease of persons over 40 years of age or _____.
7. Insulin directly stimulates the synthesis of storage lipid within the fat cell, blocks the breakdown and release of stored lipid, promotes _____ acid uptake, and directly stimulates protein synthetic processes.
8. Significant metabolic derangements _____ when insulin action is lost.
9. Common _____ symptoms of diabetes mellitus result from osmotic and metabolic changes.
10. Ketoacidosis is primarily seen in patients with IDDM who have little or no endogenous insulin production; these patients are called ketosis-_____ diabetics.

L	L	G	A	E
U	I	O	N	R
B	U	P	O	S
S	R	I	I	D
C	L	A	S	D

11. _____   14. _____

12. _____   15. _____

13. _____

11. Patients with NIDDM who produce enough insulin to suppress _____ breakdown are resistant to ketosis.
12. Pathologic changes in _____ vessels, nerves, and kidneys occur in diabetic patients.
13. Pathologic changes may be delayed or reduced in severity by strict control of the blood _____ level from the earliest possible time after the appearance of diabetes.
14. Testing for glucose in _____ (glucosuria) is one diagnostic procedure to screen for diabetes mellitus.
15. The drug _____ sulfonylureas are oral hypoglycemic agents useful only in patients who produce some insulin on their own.

Medication Cards

These sample medication cards have been printed on the front and back of this page so they can be easily reproduced for clinical use. We recommend they be photocopied double-sided and cut in 4" by 6" cards.

Drug Name: _____ Trade Name: _____
Major Drug Category: _____
Drug Action: _____
_____

Uses: _____
_____

Side Effects/Adverse Reactions: _____
_____

Significant Drug Interactions: _____
_____

Usual Drug Dosage: _____
Nursing Management:
Assessment: _____
Intervention: _____
Education: _____
Evaluation: _____

Drug Name: _____ Trade Name: _____
Major Drug Category: _____
Drug Action: _____
_____

Uses: _____
_____

Side Effects/Adverse Reactions: _____
_____

Significant Drug Interactions: _____
_____

Usual Drug Dosage: _____
Nursing Management:
Assessment: _____
Intervention: _____
Education: _____
Evaluation: _____

Client ID   Diagnosis   Comments Re: Administration/Client Response

_____

_____

_____

_____

_____

_____

_____

_____

_____

Client ID   Diagnosis   Comments Re: Administration/Client Response

_____

_____

_____

_____

_____

_____

_____

_____

_____

Medication Cards

These sample medication cards have been printed on the front and back of this page so they can be easily reproduced for clinical use. We recommend they be photocopied double-sided and cut in 4" by 6" cards.

Drug Name: _____ Trade Name: _____
Major Drug Category: _____
Drug Action: _____
_____
Uses: _____
_____
Side Effects/Adverse Reactions: _____
_____
Significant Drug Interactions:_____
_____
Usual Drug Dosage: _____
Nursing Management:
Assessment: _____
Intervention: _____
Education: _____
Evaluation:_____

Drug Name: _____ Trade Name: _____
Major Drug Category: _____
Drug Action: _____
_____
Uses: _____
_____
Side Effects/Adverse Reactions: _____
_____
Significant Drug Interactions:_____
_____
Usual Drug Dosage: _____
Nursing Management:
Assessment: _____
Intervention: _____
Education: _____
Evaluation:_____

Client ID   Diagnosis   Comments Re: Administration/Client Response

Client ID   Diagnosis   Comments Re: Administration/Client Response

Medication Cards

These sample medication cards have been printed on the front and back of this page so they can be easily reproduced for clinical use. We recommend they be photocopied double-sided and cut in 4" by 6" cards.

Drug Name: _____ Trade Name: _____
Major Drug Category: _____
Drug Action: _____
_____

Uses: _____
_____

Side Effects/Adverse Reactions: _____
_____

Significant Drug Interactions:_____
_____

Usual Drug Dosage: _____
Nursing Management:
Assessment: _____
Intervention: _____
Education: _____
Evaluation:_____

Drug Name: _____ Trade Name: _____
Major Drug Category: _____
Drug Action: _____
_____

Uses: _____
_____

Side Effects/Adverse Reactions: _____
_____

Significant Drug Interactions:_____
_____

Usual Drug Dosage: _____
Nursing Management:
Assessment: _____
Intervention: _____
Education: _____
Evaluation:_____

Client ID   Diagnosis   Comments Re: Administration/Client Response

Client ID   Diagnosis   Comments Re: Administration/Client Response